FASTING
CAN SAVE
YOUR LIFE

Other books by Herbert M. Shelton about fasting

Fasting for Renewal of Life

The Science and Fine Art of Fasting

HERBERT M. SHELTON

FASTING CAN SAVE YOUR LIFE

Natural Hygiene Press

FIRST EDITION, JULY 1964
SECOND PRINTING, MARCH 1965
THIRD PRINTING, JUNE 1967
FOURTH PRINTING, DECEMBER 1973
FIFTH PRINTNG, DECEMBER 1975
SECOND EDITION, DECEMBER 1978
SECOND PRINTING, FEBRUARY 1980
THIRD PRINTING, MAY 1981

ISBN 0-914532-23-5

Library of Congress Catalog Number: 78-70060

PRINTED IN THE UNITED STATES OF AMERICA

BOOK PUBLISHING DIVISION OF ANHS
NON-PROFIT, NON-SECTARIAN, TAX EXEMPT
NATURAL HYGIENE PRESS
698 BROOKLAWN AVE., BRIDGEPORT, CT. 06004

Dedication

To the millions of sufferers who are agonizing through their lives in search of health and not knowing where or how to find it, in the firm conviction, born of years of practical experience in the application of fasting to the problems of health, that fasting and a *Hygienic* way of life will lead to vigorous health, this book is dedicated by the author.

Contents

FASTING CAN SAVE YOUR LIFE

Preface to the Second Edition

Much water, much of it dirty, has passed under the bridge since the first edition of *Fasting Can Save Your Life* came from the press. Many newspaper and magazine articles and several books on fasting have been published presenting such a wide variety of contradictory views and opinions that the reading public is hopelessly confused. The greater part of this mass of contradictory material has revolved about the propriety or impropriety of the use of the fast as a means of reducing weight. A large part of it has stressed the largely imaginary dangers of fasting. Much of it has emphasized the demand that any fast of more than three days' duration should be done under medical supervision, preferably in a hsopital. Some of the books and articles have presented the reader with "just as good" or better substitutes for the fast. There is also much disagreement about the proper conduct of the fast. When the experts disagree so widely what is the poor reader to do?

One "scientific" experimenter adds greatly to the confusion by his use, several times in the course of a short article, of the phrase *starvation therapy*. Several of the men of *science* use the terms *fasting* and *starvation* synonymously, whereas the simple truth is that if one is fasting, one is not starving and if one is starving, one is not fasting. The loose use of the terms fasting and starving as of identical meaning and the implied assumption that the two processes are identical, when this is not done with the deliberate intent of arousing prejudice, is a reliable index of the confusion in the mind of the writer.

The phrases "untoward side effects" and "adverse reactions" appear so often in the writings of scientific experimenters that, when reading them, one easily gets the idea that one is reading about drugs. When a fast is entered and the faster abstains from tea, coffee, alcohol, soda fountain slops, condiments, spices, mustard, food additives and other irritating and stimulating substances which he is accustomed to taking both with his meals and between meals, and discontinues dosing himself at intervals with aspirin or other drugs, he experiences headache, dizziness, weakness, trembling, pains in the abdomen, back, and joints; he may faint; and he

11

may be nauseous and even vomit. These "withdrawal symptoms" are not "side effects" of fasting, but are the extensions of the same symptoms, with which he was annoyed while eating and which he smothered with frequent cigarettes, cups of coffee, Tums or other popular drug-desserts. That these so-called "side effects" of fasting are not caused by fasting, but by the habitual poisoning indulged in as a regular part of his daily life, is shown by the fact that if the fast is continued the symptoms all clear up.

Another cause of "untoward side-effects" is the practice of the scientific experimenters of encouraging fasters to supply their need for fluid (water) by drinking tea, coffee, soda fountain slop, beer, wine, ale, and strained soups or broth. There are the additional practices of giving drugs to suppress every discomfort that may arise and of permitting the continuance of smoking or other drug taking.

There is a great difference between a poisoned fast and an unpoisoned one. Not until the scientific men test the unpoisoned fast will they be in a position to properly evaluate the results of fasting. To put a very fat woman on a fast and continue it for over three hundred days all the while supplying her fluid needs with tea and coffee, both of them containing the heart irritant caffeine, and blaming the impairment of the heart upon the fast and not upon the caffeine, does not make good sense. Likewise, dosing the faster with liberal quantities of synthetic vitamins and drug-store minerals ruinously affects the whole experiment.

All together too much emphasis has been placed upon the dangers of protein deficiency, thus creating great fear of fasting. The evils of protein deficiencies conjured up out of the void have frightened great numbers of people. There is no danger of protein deficiency developing in a fast of ordinary duration. It is perhaps a possibility in a fast of two to three hundred days or more, but the greatest danger in these extremely long fasts lies in the poisons taken as drink and as medicine.

It will be difficult to fully assess the physiological wreakage that results from the repeated examinations and testing that constitute an important feature of the hospital-supervision of the fast. The depressing effect of daily pulse-counting, blood-pressure taking, heart examination, blood and urine sampling, checking the temperature and similar psychologically disturbing activities is considerable. For best results, the faster needs calm, quiet, cheerful surroundings. The faster needs to relax and take life easy. Too much officious meddling is ruinous to poise. Poise is also disturbed by the practice of keeping the thought always in the faster's mind that death is imminent.

To add to the prevailing confusion, an effort is being made to revive the old enema practices. To this end there has been a repetition of the old fallacies about reabsorption of waste from the colon. In all of the discussion of this subject, I have never seen one reference to the fact that the faster's bowels act when there is a need for action. There may actually develop a diarrhea.

Advocates of the enema warn of serious complications that may arise out of the autointoxications resulting from reabsorption of waste matter thrown into the colon. This is certain evidence that the man uttering the warning has never observed a fast in which no enema was used, else he would know how false are his warnings.

Finally, there are those who contend that a period on fruit or fruit juice or vegetable juice produces the same or greater beneficial results than the fast. They call the period on fruit or juice a fruit fast or a juice fast, whereas, in sober reality, the period on fruit or on juice is more likely to be a fruit feast or a juice feast. For example, when on a grape diet one is urged to eat large quantities of grapes. When on a carrot juice diet, one is urged to drink large quantities of carrot juice. The promoter of wheat grass juice therapy is emphatic in her assertion that the "wheat grass juice fast" is superior to abstinence from all food, or what they persist in designating a water fast.

This misuse of language is exceeded only by the physicians who use the phrase *therapeutic starvation*. The word starvation means the process of dying because of lack of some essential of life, such as warmth, water, or food. The process of dying would seem to be a very poor therapeutic process.

The juice diets have their legitimate places in the life of the *Hygienist*. We would make a serious mistake, however, should we rule out the total fast and rely heavily upon juice diets. Fasting is a biological process and belongs to the world of life.

Herbert M. Shelton
San Antonio, Texas
June 1978

Preface to the First Edition

Few subjects going back in mankind's history are so widely misunderstood, in our modern, high-caloric civilization, as fasting. The important role it can play, and has played, is often distorted in the public mind, or twisted out of shape by grotesque and groundless fears, based not on truth but on prejudices, scientific misinformation or complete lack of information.

The purpose of this book, based upon my own experiences, studies and observations over a period of forty-five years of conducting fasts as a *Hygienist*, is to put into focus the true role fasting can play in promoting and maintaining good health, in eliminating pain, in weight reduction and control, and in prolonging human life.

This role will be explained and discussed in detail, not as a *cure*, for fasting itself is not a *cure*, but as a means of permitting the resources of the body itself to take over, to effect healing, or take off pounds at a rate unmatched by any other method.

One of the primary purposes of this book is to answer the many questions about fasting which have begun to flood the offices of those who write about weight problems for the newspapers and magazines. Since overeating and overweight have become primary health problems in the United States and some European countries, the quest for information about how to lose pounds safely is a never-ending one on the modern scene.

At the same time a revival of interest in the means of mind-body care as developed by those who believe in *Natural Hygiene* has brought close attention to the theories and findings of *Hygienists* developed over nearly a century and a half.

It is axiomatic that the medical profession has battled stoutly all these theories. Many of the advances of recent decades have been achieved only after bitter warfare and denunciation by entrenched medical opinions.

Progress has been made inch by inch—spoonful by spoonful—in the business of developing proper eating and living habits. Yet fasting goes back over the centuries—not only in matters of health, but also in religious ritual.

15

In recent years investigators who have contributed greatly are Dr. Henry S. Tanner, Sylvester Graham, Dr. Robert Walter, Dr. John H. Tilden and Dr. George S. Weger.

One could multiply these names many times over. These are the experienced men of the nineteenth and twentieth centuries—scientists, investigators, scholars who dedicated themselves to the study and practice of the basic truths of *Hygienic* living with particular emphasis on the role of the fast.

It must be understood that for the best results, it is unwise to departmentalize too much in our thinking. The body is a complex organism in which all parts are interrelated. Good health therefore is a single thing, encompassing and including every aspect of ourselves—physical, mental and emotional. What we are considering here goes beyond any simple problems. It concerns the whole individual.

These are general considerations presenting an approach to good living. Only the expert in fasting is capable of directing the individual with his particular health problem, his special need and goal. Our purpose here is to give the layman, the average reader, a broad perspective with some details and occasionally technical background information and hope, in an area that has to do with ways by which man can live better, feel better—last longer.

Because overeating has become one of the great physiological and psychological problems of our age here in America, I am placing particular importance on this aspect of the subject in the early chapters of this book. Weight reduction alone is only one part of the picture. To maintain proper weight and proper physical condition, many of us require a total renovation of our eating habits, our working habits, our understanding of the real need for rest and relaxation. All of these are a part of the broad philosophy embodied in the chapters of this book.

There is no necessity to be overweight, nor any need to be crippled with self-inflicted disease brought on by the totality of destructive living habits which too many of us pursue.

I am not therefore presenting merely the *Hygienic* concepts of diet, exercise, rest, correct habits and routines. For the present indeed, I will deal with a totally new way of life.

Herbert M. Shelton

1
Fasting and You!

Fasting is much more than simply not eating: it is both a science and an art. It has meaning in terms of overall well-being and affects the psychological and emotional aspects of our lives.

Fasting, as we use the term here, means total abstinence from all food for a definite period of time. The word comes from the old English word *faesten*, which means firm or fixed. In other words, the fast is something we hold to on a firm basis under controlled and fixed conditions.

In religious terms it may mean abstinence from certain food on certain holy days. But this is partial abstinence rather than total abstinence. I know persons who have "fasted" during Lent and actually gained weight rather than lost, because they substituted for the dishes they gave up foods which put on even more pounds.

Those who think that fasting is equivalent to starvation are entirely wrong. There are basically two periods in the process of abstaining from food that should concern us here—the *fasting* period proper and the period of *starvation*.

As we study the phenomena of abstinence in greater detail, the distinction between these two phases will become clear. From the outset however, it is essential to understand that the fasting stage continues so long as the body supports itself on the stored reserves within its tissues. Starvation begins when abstinence is carried beyond the time when these stored reserves are used up or have dropped to a dangerously low level.

We must understand also that there is much loose terminology that adds to confusion on the subject of fasting. For example: we hear people speak of going on a "water fast" which technically would imply that they were giving up drinking water. What they mean, actually, is that they are going on a fast in which they give up everything but water. The same illogicality exists in the expression, "going on a fruit juice fast" or a "vegetable juice fast." Again what is meant is that they are giving up everything *except* fruit or vegetable juice.

The term "partial fast" is used for any form of fasting where individuals put extremely limiting conditions on what they eat. The misuse of the word *"starving,"* not only in the vernacular, but even in some scientific papers, has done vast harm. The word is derived from the Anglo-Saxon *stearfan*, which means to die, not only from lack of food but also from overall exposure to cold. This is how the phrase "starving cold" developed.

Starvation is a process of dying, in effect. You cannot starve yourself into good health. You can fast for proper and reasonable periods and thereby improve your physical condition and often restore yourself to good health. It is possible to abstain from food for long periods of time with beneficial effects. At the point where the experienced advisor who conducts the fast realizes that the second phase of abstention from food is imminent, the fast is broken.

I have said the fast is part of a new way of life which I outline in this book. Thus it is not used only to lose weight. It can be and certainly is equally important as a part of the function of maintaining or even restoring good health.

The sick or wounded animal finds a secluded spot where he can keep warm, where he is protected from the weather, where he can have peace and quiet and be undisturbed. There he rests and fasts. He may, for example, have lost a limb, but he lies there in his privacy and generally recovers without drugs, without bandages or surgery.

In the animal world fasting is a tremendously important factor of existence. Animals fast not only when sick or wounded but also during hibernation or aestivation (sleeping throughout the summer in tropical climates).

Some animals fast during the mating season and in many cases during the nursing period. Some birds fast while their eggs are being hatched. Some animals fast immediately after birth. There are forms of spiders who do not eat for six months after they are born. Some wild creatures fast when taken into captivity, and a domestic pet, a dog, or a cat, may not eat for several days when it comes into a new environment. Animals also survive forced fasts during periods of drought, snow, cold, and live for long periods when no food is available.

In mankind fasting has been practised in various parts of the world over centuries for religious reasons, for self-discipline, for political purposes and as a means of restoring health. Only in recent centuries has the concept that we must eat to keep up our strength become a deeply entrenched idea. Dr. Felix Oswald, a Dutch physician who came to America before the turn of the century, declares: "The fast cure method is not limited to our dumb fellow creatures. It is a common experience that pain, fever, gastric congestion and even mental afflictions take away the appetite and only unwise nurses will try to thwart the purposes of Nature in this respect."

Fasting is centuries old; we read of it in the Bible and in Homer. It was employed in the care of the sick in ancient temples in Egypt, Greece and throughout the Mediterranean world. The use of the fast in acute disease dates back to remote times.

It was prescribed by Arabian physicians during the long dark night of Europe's Medieval Age. In Italy, Neapolitan physicians as long ago as one hundred and fifty years, employed fasts that sometimes lasted for forty days in the case of fever patients.

This writer has been engaged in conducting fasts since the summer of 1920. In this period of approximately forty-five years, I have conducted thousands of fasts ranging from a few days duration to ninety days, both for weight reduction and in connection with helping the body recover from physical impairment.

One particular case of an elderly man is of special interest because the results were so successful.

Mr. A.B. was seventy years of age and had been sick a large part of those years. For thirteen years he had suffered with bronchial asthma and during this time he had been hospitalized five times. For an even longer time he had suffered with sinus trouble. For six years he had been completely deaf in his left ear, while he had suffered with an enlarged prostate gland for more than six years and had been impotent for a few years. He wore glasses, was bald headed, and had the usual "minor symptoms" that indicate the condition of his organism was not good, although it is common to ignore these evidences of incipient disease.

Although he had been treated by the usual methods over the years, he had realized no genuine benefits from this care. Like others who suffer as he did, he grew from bad to worse. It is generally known that the regular care of asthmatics is purely palliative and that the patient commonly grows progressively worse with the passage of time. It is equally well known that the regular modes of care fail to do more than provide doubtful temporary relief for the sufferer with sinus disease. It seems hardly necessary to add that nothing of real value is done for deafness and for enlargement of the prostate gland. All of these conditions are commonly understood to be *incurable*.

Leaving his hospital bed in Chicago, the fifth time he was hospitalized for asthma, Mr. A.B. went directly to the airport and boarded a plane going south and went to a place that was reputed to be very successful in its care of asthma sufferers. Still wheezing, he was uncertain that he could make the trip, but had determined to try. His own statement was that he had suffered enough and that he was convinced that the regular methods of care offered him no real promise of health. Like many thousands of other asthmatics, he had given the regular plans of care every opportunity to free him effectively of his suffering and they had failed him.

Arriving at the institution in the southwest, he was admitted and told that he would have to discontinue at once and thereafter all drugs that he had been using for relief. "But," he asked, "what shall I do if I have an attack of asthma?"

"You will grit your teeth and clench your fists and suffer through it," was the reply. "You cannot get well if you continue to use drugs."

He was sent to bed and instructed to remain there and take nothing into his mouth but water until he was told that he could resume eating. The treatment is going to be worse than the disease, he thought. Could he go without food? He was weak from years of suffering and from a lengthy period during which he was unable to secure enough oxygen. He was assured that he would be carefully watched and that no harm would befall him.

With a certain amount of trepidation he entered upon what was to be a new and surprisingly pleasant experience. Fasting is not always a pleasant experience, but it can be a very interesting and even highly pleasurable experience. The freedom and ease that one experiences during a period of abstinence from food often enables one to discover new and previously undreamed-of depths of meaning to life.

About four o'clock in the morning of his first night of fasting, Mr. A.B. developed a severe paroxysm of asthma. He was unable to breathe while lying in bed, so he sat up on the side of the bed and rang for assistance. The doctor came and after observing and examining him, said: "You'll be all right in a brief time. It will take about twenty-four hours for you to become free of asthmatic symptoms, and then you'll be comfortable."

When the doctor left, Mr. A.B. was struggling for air. "What kind of a place have I come to," Mr. A.B. asked the man in the next bed. "They won't even do anything to relieve me of my attack." He continued to struggle for air for a few more minutes, then relief came and he fell asleep.

When the doctor saw him again in the morning, Mr. A.B. was feeling so well that he was ready to forgive the seeming neglect of the latter part of the night. He was more than overjoyed when he went on day after day breathing as easily as when he was a small boy, with not the slightest sign of asthma. He had not another single paroxysm of asthma so long as he remained at the institution. His sinuses were still draining and the fast was continued. After about six days without food, he was able to void urine as freely as a boy. His prostate gland had shrunken to nearly normal size.

He continued to fast and watched a day by day disappearance of symptoms, until his sinuses cleared up, his breathing was a pleasure and his chest was a source of real joy. On the twenty-fifth day of the fast, he asked the doctor if he could not break the fast. He was informed that this would be premature, that he was not fully recovered and that it would be wise to continue. "You are not in jail," said the doctor. "You cannot be made to fast against your will. But, if you want my best advice you will continue for a while."

He took the doctor's advice and went ahead with the fast. What will always seem to him as a miracle was the fact that on the thirty-sixth day of the fast, he regained his hearing in his deaf ear. His hearing was so good that he could easily hear the low ticking of a small watch when held at arm's length from his ear. Equally important is the fact that the recovery of hearing was permanent. The fast was continued through the forty-second day and then feeding was resumed.

But he had another surprise in store for him. He discovered, upon his return home, a few weeks after the fast was broken, that he was no longer impotent. As restoration of potency in men and overcoming of frigidity in women are not uncommon results of the fast, this was no surprise to the head of the institution.

This is no fanciful case, but an actual account of the recovery of a man who had suffered as I have described and who underwent the fast, as I have here portrayed it, and who made the recovery that has been pictured. It was not an unusual case, except in the variety of conditions that he suffered with, unless we say that the recovery of hearing is not a rule when the deaf undergo a fast. It is only an occasional result of fasting. This is so because deafness, like loss of vision, may be due to a variety of abnormal conditions of the ear, and not all of them are remediable. Blindness is only occasionally recoverable by fasting for the same reason, although restoration of good vision, in errors of refraction, is not at all uncommon.

The dramatic recoveries that occur during a fast of proper length and taken under the most favorable conditions can be believed only by those who have had opportunity to observe them. The general tendency of both the layman and the physician, when hearing stories of such recoveries, is to dismiss them as too fantastic for consideration. Yet, there is nothing miraculous about the effects of the fast. If we think on the matter a little, we cannot escape the conclusion that fasting is the most natural and the most sensible means of care of the sick body of which we have any knowledge.

For over one hundred and forty years, natural *Hygienists* have employed the fast as a means of promoting health and enabling the body to recover speedily from illness. They have amassed extraordinary clinical experience in this area. These experiences turn into the deeply-rooted conviction that the fast is a constructive force which must be utilized and developed as part of the regular practices of modern life.

There are, of course, critics of fasting. Most of them know very little about fasting, or its techniques. A. Rabogliati, A.M., M.D., F.R.C.S., of England so well puts it: "The most popular criticisms of fasting are written by people who have never missed a meal in their lives."

Whether it is to maintain or to restore good health, to gain weight or to lose weight the role of fasting is a vital factor that can no longer be overlooked by any who are concerned with personal health and well-being—mentally and physically.

2

Pounds that Slip Away

The big business of losing weight, figure control, diet-in-comfort plans and similar programs have developed into one of the great industries of our age. Everyone considers himself an expert. Fad diets range for a few months and give way to the next crash wonder. This week it is an ice cream diet. The next it is bananas. The week after that a protein diet, nothing but juicy steaks. Eat yourself *thin!*

Overweight is becoming an increasingly perplexing problem, not alone for adult men and women, but for children also. Several facts are responsible for this, but, in general, we may say that the increased abundance of food, together with the increased income of the American people, on the one hand, and the changes in work resulting from the shortened work-day, shortened work-week, modern transportation and the many labor-saving devices that take much of the burden off the shoulders of men and women, have resulted in the increase of weight. Just at a time when our reduced labors have reduced our need for food, increased production, artificially increased palatability and increased income have served to increase our food consumption.

Hygienists are realists. Nothing can circumvent the fact that the quickest, surest, safest way to lose weight is by fasting, and the surest way of maintaining the proper weight level is by refusing to return to the wrong eating habits.

The disappointingly slow method of losing weight by "going on a diet" is rarely very successful for the reason that it is a long-drawn-out process requiring more self-control and a much longer period of control than the average person is capable of. A not uncommon outcome of such programs is that, after a brief period, during which time a few pounds are lost, the obese individual returns to his prior overeating and puts back all the weight lost, and often additional pounds. Only rarely does one see an obese individual stick to a reducing diet for a prolonged period.

To begin with, as I have stated in many lectures, and will continue to remind the reader, do not enter upon a fast on your own without the guidance of an expert in the field of conducting fasts. While fasting is perfectly safe as a health and weight reducing measure, it does involve the complex human organism, and it should be watched over and directed at all times by a qualified person who knows what he may expect, or what trouble signs to watch for during the fast.

How much can one expect to lose? The loss rate of course varies with the individual, but the average for a protracted fast runs around two and one-half pounds a day. Is this heavy weight loss safe? It is as long as it is conducted under proper controls and with proper and continuing rest.

Let me cite here briefly the most striking advantages of fasting for weight reduction:

1. Safe rapid loss is registered on the fast.

2. The fast is far more pleasant than the reducing diet—the nagging desire to eat is missing.

3. Weight loss may be secured without resulting in flabbiness or sagging of the skin and tissues. However, this is not true of elderly persons.

When the overweight individual undergoes a marked reduction of weight, several indications of improved health follow immediately:

1. Breathing is freer.

2. There is greater ease of movement.

3. There is loss of "that tired feeling."

4. There is a disappearance of the sense of fullness and discomfort in the abdomen.

5. Symptoms of indigestion cease to annoy.

6. Other discomforts cease.

7. Blood pressure is lowered and the load the heart has to carry is lessened.

All of these evidences of benefit are noticeable, but the improvements are commonly out of all proportion to the weight lost, thus indicating that reduction of the amount of food eaten itself resulted in improved health. There is every reason for thinking that the greatly reduced intake of sugar, starches and fat and the over-all reduction of the amount of food eaten is beneficial.

In 1962, a woman began a fast to reduce weight under my guidance. At the conclusion she told me: "It has been an amazing experience: the pleasure of seeing those pounds melt away. I never saw fat go so fast." Another woman remarked after a fast of fifteen days undertaken for reducing: "I was at a well-advertised health spa. They kept me on a diet of seven hundred calories a day. I was hungry all the time. This fast has been a pleasure."

A third woman said after a week of fasting to lose pounds: "This has been the most remarkable experience of my life. I have enjoyed this fast and rest. I never knew before that people fast, but I have enjoyed it."

Are these expressions typical? Hardly. Fasting is not always the pleasant experience these women found it to be, but it is rarely disagreeable enough to justify discontinuing it until one's goal has been attained. But it is frequently a far more pleasurable experience than many people have in their daily eating habits. In many conditions of life, every meal is followed by discomforts and even actual pain. In these states, the fast is often such a relief that it becomes a joy.

There is always great satisfaction in watching the fat melt away at the rate of two to four pounds a day. To lose nineteen pounds in a week is a highly pleasing experience (there are exceptions in which the weight loss is not so great) for the first several days of the fast. The rate of loss is not uniform and there are periods when the scales register no loss for a day or two at a time. The rapid loss registered at the beginning of the fast does not continue throughout the whole of a long fast.

Not only is there safety in fasting for weight reduction, there is also greater ease than there is in dieting. One reason for this is that unlike almost all dieters, the faster is not hungry all the time. His taste buds are not constantly tempting him. The flood of gastric juices is not being constantly activated.

The faster may experience some desire for food during the first or second day of the fast or may not desire food at all. Hunger subsides usually by the end of the third day. And unless the fast is broken for some reason, the faster can continue without experiencing either weakness or hunger.

I state these facts out of my own personal experience but they are also verified by investigations. Two series of experiments carried out by regular medical men in accredited hospitals, have developed empirical evidence sufficient to satisfy the experimenter scientifically that fasting is not only a safe and speedy way of reducing weight, but is also the most comfortable way of reducing.

One of these experiments was carried out by Lyon Bloom, M.D., in the Piedmont Hospital in Atlanta, Georgia, where he conducted a lengthy series of experiments on fasting in reducing weight. This was followed up by Garfield Duncan, M.D., of the University of Pennsylvania, who is regarded as an authority on weight reduction and whose independent tests include Bloom's findings and conclusions.

These two medical investigators found that fasting men lose an average of 2.6 pounds a day, while women fasters lose an average of 2.7 pounds a day. Both Bloom and Duncan confirm that the fasters were not hungry. Instead they reported an amazing absence of hunger with no apparent mental or physical strain. One of the fasters was quoted as saying: "I feel better than ever before in my life." A woman faster, after forty-eight hours without food, volunteered the information that she was not half so hungry as she used to be after missing a single meal.

Bloom is quoted, from the summary of the experiments: "The present preoccupation with eating at regular intervals leads to the misconception that fasting is unpleasant." He stated further, that, in his opinion, as the result of the findings of these tests, fasting is well tolerated by the human system provided there is free access to water.

In a later series of experiments, Bloom permitted a faster to go four consecutive weeks without food, with no ill effects. In reading his report of experiments to the 111th Annual Meeting of the American Medical Association, Duncan declared: "Although short periods of total fasting may seem barbaric, this method of reduction is marvelously well tolerated." He added that we have evidence that these obese persons fully enjoyed the total fasting periods, due probably in part to their elation that hunger is not a problem while major reductions in weight are being accomplished.

Both men reported that in longer fasts the weight loss levels off to about a pound a day. Bloom stated fasting has also proved to be an extremely effective method of weight control.

In the healthy individual, fasting only to lose weight, I do not insist on rest in bed, but permit considerable exercise—even at times giving a prescribed course of physical workouts. This does not increase the rate of loss as much as one might expect, but it does assist in retaining the tone of the tissues.

The amount of exercise required to reduce weight by exercise alone is far more than the average person is willing to undertake and more than many of them should undergo. To lose one pound of fat requires playing twenty-three holes of golf, sawing wood for ten and one-half hours, riding a horse for approximately forty-three miles.

Exercise always has the added hazard of increasing the appetite. During the fast it should be controlled and used only to the extent that the adviser feels desirable for the individual undergoing the fasting process.

While there are varying rates of metabolism, my experience indicates that most overweight is due, not to glandular disorders but to habitual overeating. There is little truth in the idea that with some people everything they eat turns to fat. The real truth is that they are eating not only more than they should, but more than they really want.

How much weight loss per day is safe in fasting? The answer here is that since fasting is total abstention, the body itself decides what rate loss is proper. When fat tissue is soft and flabby, weight is usually lost rapidly in the early days of the fast. I have seen losses ranging from four to six pounds a day in fasting. The loss of twenty pounds in a week is not at all difficult in a great many cases.

With those who have a very low rate of metabolism, the rate of loss from the outset of the fast is slow—at times even disappointingly so. Let me reiterate once more, any fasting of more than a few days should be done only under experienced supervision. In all cases where there is any organic defect or chronic ailment, such as heart disease or blood deficiency, even the shortest fast should be supervised. Again let me say there is no essential danger in fasting but one must be properly safeguarded against any danger from hidden conditions that might reveal themselves when no food is taken.

I cite the possibility in order to give the rounded picture of fasting. Let me reassure the reader, however, that such dangers are rare. If the reader is in good health, if he follows the proper procedures under proper experienced guidance, the fast should be for him not only a way of losing poundage, but an exhilarating and exciting adventure, the beginning of a new way of thinking about himself.

3

Living without Eating

In March, 1963, newspapers around the world described the almost incredible story of the seven weeks deprivation of food and the survival of Ralph Flores, a forty-two year old pilot of San Bruno, California, and twenty-one-year old Helen Klaben, a co-ed of Brooklyn, New York, following a plane crash on a mountain side in Northern British Columbia. The couple was rescued March 25, 1963, after forty-nine days in the wilderness in the dead of winter, over thirty days of this time without any food at all.

By means of a fire, a lean-to and heavy clothes in which they wrapped themselves, they managed to withstand the bitter cold. During the first four days after the crash, Helen Klaben ate four tins of sardines, two tins of fruit and some crackers. Twenty days after the crash, the pair took their last "food"—two tubes of toothpaste. Melted snow became their diet, for breakfast, lunch and the evening meal. "For the last six weeks," she explained, "we lived on water. We drank it three ways: hot, cold and boiled." Varying it in this way helped reduce the monotony of their single item menu of snow.

Miss Klaben who was "pleasingly plump" at the time of the plane crash, was happily surprised, at the ordeal's end, to learn that her weight loss totalled thirty pounds.

Flores, who was more active during their enforced fast, had lost forty pounds. Physicians who examined them after the rescue, found them to be in "remarkably good" condition.

Many thousands of men and women have gone without food for much longer periods, not only without harm, but with positive benefits. Periods of abstinence under such taxing conditions as the ones these two people endured and survived are extremely rare.

Whatever our view of the origins of life, we must all recognize the fact that nature provides for need, including provision for plants and animals over periods of food scarcity. Famine is more frequent in nature than we commonly realize. Winter, floods, periods of drought, often leave wild animals less well fed and watered than domestic animals who can generally depend upon their masters to store food for continuous food supplies. In the wild state, both herbivorous and carnivorous animals often subsist on reduced food supplies. Most wild dogs are gaunt: like the dogs, lean, hungry wolves whose skeletons have shrunk with their bowels, are common; "half-starved" wild cattle and horses were once common. What happens to these creatures under such stringent conditions? Do they die of starvation? The answer is they rarely do.

In his *Zoological Sketches*, Dr. Felix L. Oswald writes: "In a sparsely settled country, animal refugees soon accustom themselves to the vicissitudes of their wild life. The ten months' drought back in 1877, which almost exterminated the domestic cattle of southern Brazil, was braved by the pampas cows, whom experience had taught to derive their water supply from bulbous roots, cactus leaves, and excavations in the moist river-sand. Solid food is only a secondary requirement.

"The Syrian Khamr dogs manage to eke out a living in regions where no human hunter would discover a trace of game and where water is as scarce as in the eternal abodes of Dives; nay, they multiply, for the Khamr bitch, like other poor mothers, is generally over-blest with progeny; six youngsters is said to be the minimum.

"A sausage-maker would probably decline to invest in Khamr dogs: the word *leanness* does not begin to describe their physical condition; *strappedness* would be more to the purpose, if an Arkansas adjective admits of that suffix—skin and sinews tightly stretched over a framework of bones. I saw their relatives in Dalmatia, and often wondered that they did not rattle when they ran; but Dalmatia is still a country of vineyards and sand rabbits, while the Syrian desert has ceased to produce thornberries. Without moisture not even a curse can bear fruit."

That animals do survive such conditions and go on generation after generation is a fact of utmost significance. A weasel hiding in a closed room will survive for days without food and seek food when released. The hibernating bear, taking no food for prolonged periods, will give birth to her cub, and secrete milk upon which it feeds. The fasting salmon and fur seal bull are very active while abstaining from food. These few examples of activity while fasting suffice to reveal that the fasting body does have means of meeting its energy requirements, even if these are at a low ebb and this is far from being true in the case of the salmon and the seal.

One of Sweden's distinguished biochemists, Dr. Ragnar Berg, a Nobel Prize winner, and an authority on nutrition, says, "One can fast a long time; we know of fasts of over a hundred days duration, so we have no need of fearing that we will die of hunger."

The actual time period of abstinence forced upon Mr. Flores and Miss Klaben was of relatively moderate duration. The question is not how long man can fast, but what are the provisions of nature that enable him to do so.

Wear and waste, repair and replenishment, are continuous and almost simultaneous processes in all living structures, and none of these processes halt during a fast. The hibernating animal in the far north must produce sufficient heat to maintain body warmth. Both man and animal, while fasting, must breathe and the heart must continue to pulsate. The blood must continue to flow and the organs of elimination must continue their work of freeing the tissues of waste. The vital functions of life must be carried on, even if at a slightly reduced rate. Cells must be replenished, wounds must be healed. All of this, as I know from years of observations, goes on during a fast, moreover, and I will cite examples of this fact later, physical development and growth may take place, even while no food is being taken.

All manifestations of life—movement, secretion, digestion, and similar processes—depend upon the use of the materials of the body. If an organ is to work, it must be supplied with the materials with which to work. In the absence of fresh supplies with which to replace those that have been used up the organ wastes and weakens. If life is to continue, a basic irreducible level of activity is imperative. Even the hibernating and aestivating animal, with activities reduced to a bare minimum consistent with continued life, must breathe and the heart must pulsate.

In the case of the bear that gives birth to a cub while hibernating and suckles it, with milk produced during hibernation, for this purpose, we have a significant example of the possibilities of the fasting animal meeting the needs of its functioning tissues from sources other than the food eaten daily. All of these activities require food, which must be supplied from some source while the animal is fasting.

An understanding of the process by which the body nourishes its vital tissues and sustains its essential functions during prolonged abstinence, and the sources upon which it draws, will help us understand how the body can survive periods when outside food is not available or cannot be digested.

The normal body provides itself with a store of nutritive materials that are put away in the form of fat, bone marrow, glycogen, muscle juices, lacteal fluids, minerals and vitamins. Always the healthy body maintains in store adequate nutritive reserves to tide it over several days, weeks or even over two or three months of lack of food. This remains true whether fasting is enforced, as in the case of a plane crash, or of entombed miners, or is brought on by illness where one cannot swallow or digest food, or by free choice as in voluntary fasting to lose weight. When food is not taken, the body draws upon its reserves with which to nourish its functioning tissues. As this reserve is used up, weight is lost.

Basic in the fasting process is the fact that our "built-in pantries" contain sufficient nutriment to hold out, in most instances, for prolonged periods, especially if they are conserved and not wasted. In the blood and lymph, in the bones, and especially in the marrow of the bones, in the fat of the body, in the liver and other glands, and even in the individual cells that make up the body, are stores of protein, fat, sugar, minerals, and vitamins which may be drawn upon during periods of scarcity or when food is not usable.

Neither animal nor man can survive prolonged abstinence from food unless he carries within himself a store of reserve food on which the body can call in emergencies. The fasting organism will not be harmed by abstinence so long as the stored reserves are adequate to meet the nutritive requirements of its functioning tissues. Even thin individuals carry a reserve of food in their tissues, to tide them over periods of abstinence. These people too, may safely fast for varying periods.

By a process known technically as *autolysis*, achieved by enzymes in the tissues, these stored reserves are made available for use by the vital tissues to which they are carried by the blood and lymph as required. Glycogen or animal starch, stored in the liver, is converted to sugar and distributed, as needed, to the tissues. It is significant that, even in prolonged fasts, no beriberi, pellagra, rickets, scurvy or other "deficiency disease" ever develops, thus showing that the reserves of the body are generally well balanced.

Fasting has been shown to improve rickets and calcium metabolism. In anemia, the number of red blood cells are increased during a fast. I have observed benefits in pellagra during a fast. The bio-chemical balance may be maintained and even restored while fasting. It is important to know this, for if it were not so, the fast would prove to be deleterious.

Numerous animal experiments have shown that underfeeding, as contrasted with overfeeding, tends to prolong life and to provide for better health. Other experiments involving fasting rather than underfeeding, have shown that fasting not only prolongs life, but results in a marked degree of regeneration and rejuvenation.

Thousands of observations of both man and animals have established the fact that when the physical organism goes without food, the tissues are called upon in the inverse order of their importance to the organism. Thus fat is the first tissue to go. The stored reserves are used up before any of the functioning tissues of the body are called upon to supply nutrients for the more vital tissues such as the brain and nerves, the heart and lungs. As it feels among its supplies for proteins, sugars, fats, minerals, and vitamins, and redistributes, utilizes and conserves these stores, the fasting organism exercises an ingenuity that seems almost superhuman.

The aggregate of tissues of the organism may be regarded as a reservoir of nutriment which it may call in any direction or to any part as needed. But these tissues are not sacrificed indiscriminately. On the contrary, wastage of those organs that are primarily essential to life is repaired by withdrawal from less essential organs of materials required by the more important ones. Many of the necessary nutritive constituents, and this is especially true of certain minerals, are vigorously retained.

Studies made on men and animals to determine losses of various tissues and organs in prolonged abstinence from food have almost all been made on organisms that have died of starvation. Starvation and fasting are two totally different stages of abstinence. It should be quite obvious that the extreme losses seen at the starvation stage of abstinence are far greater than they are in a fast of reasonable length. Extreme weight losses are not experienced in any normal fast. Where they occur, the fast should be broken.

One must differentiate between fasting and starving. To *fast* is to abstain from food while one possesses adequate reserves to nourish his vital tissues; to *starve* is to abstain from food after his reserves have been exhausted so that vital tissues are sacrificed. We are not left unwarned as to when the reserves are nearing exhaustion. Hunger returns with an intensity that drives one to seek food, although during the fast proper, there is no desire for food. This differentiation between *fasting* and *starving* should help to dispel any notion that starvation sets in with the omission of the first meal.

Contrary to popular and even professional opinion, the vital tissues of a fasting organism, those tissues doing the actual work of life, do not begin to break down the instant a fast is instituted. The fasting body does lose weight, but this loss, for an extended period, is one of reserves and not of organized tissues. There are numerous examples in nature of continued growth while fasting, both of the organism as a whole and of parts that have been lost. Experiments have shown that calves continue to grow while fasting. The starfish may grow a new stomach, new tube feet, and new arms while fasting. The fasting salamander that had lost a tail, will grow a new tail while taking no food. Such facts bear out dramatically the underlying truth: the process of fasting does not suspend the constructive processes of life, but that these continue in a remarkable manner.

The efficiency of the living organism in regulating the expenditure of its resources during a fast is one of the marvels of life.

In periods of abstinence, the less important organs of the human being although they waste consequent upon the withdrawal of substance from them with which to nourish the more vital tissues, do not undergo degeneration until the starvation phase of the period of abstinence is reached. The atrophy of muscles may be no greater than that seen to occur from a lengthy period of physical inactivity, while there is no loss of muscle cells. The cells grow smaller, the fat is removed from the muscles, but the muscle retains its integrity and a surprising amount of strength.

Loss of weight varies according to the character and quality of the tissues of the individual, the amount of physical and emotional activity engaged in, and the temperature surrounding the faster. Physical activity, emotional stress, cold and poor tissues all provide for more rapid loss. Fat is lost faster than any of the other tissues of the body.

Bodily condition is, perhaps, the chief determiner of how long one may safely fast. In the case of the two who survived the plane crash, and went four weeks without food, for example, they had snow which is water and this kept them from the danger of dehydration. They could live without food; the lack of water would have been fatal. Voluntary or involuntary, the faster must have water.

It is clear then that fasting must be carried out intelligently, with proper precaution, and with common sense.

Precisely as a novice swimmer would seek expert guidance and advice before starting on a long swim, so the inexperienced faster must obtain reliable guidance as a precautionary measure before launching upon a fast of any extended duration.

4

Hunger versus Appetite

Many efforts have been made to explain the mechanism by which the sense of hunger is produced, but none has been satisfactory. In my opinion, for higher animals at least, there can be no doubt that hunger is felt through the nervous system, but this is at best a general statement. What the sensation of hunger actually is has been the subject of much speculation. For all practical purposes here, it is necessary for us primarily to distinguish between the genuine sensation of hunger and the many other sensations that are often mistaken for hunger.

Unfortunately, too many physiological investigations into hunger are limited to studies of short periods without food, a few days at the most, not enough to give a clear picture of the manner in which the body's demand for food manifests itself. It is interesting to note that trained physiologists still describe hunger in most cases in almost pathological terminology.

Hunger is a sense of distress or discomfort in the region of the stomach. It may be an actual pain. It expresses itself in hunger pangs. It is a gnawing in the stomach, an "all gone" feeling, a sense of weakness—all these are part of the popular mythology of hunger. Even headache is sometimes mistaken for hunger, and even by some trained practitioners.

The truth is that hunger is a normal, not an abnormal, sensation and all normal sensations are pleasant. It is an error to think of hunger in the terms of symptoms of disease, just as it would be to think of thirst, or any other of the body's normal desires, as painful or uncomfortable. Normal hunger is indicated by a general bodily condition—a universal call for food—, which is localized, so far as localization takes place, in the mouth, nose and throat, just as is the sense of thirst. There are no "hunger pangs" associated with *genuine* hunger; there is only a pleasant sensation in the nose, mouth and throat and a watering of the mouth. The hungry person is conscious of a desire for food, not of pain or irritation.

It is a false appetite that manifests itself by morbid irritation, *gnawing* in the stomach, pain, the feeling of weakness, and various emotionally rooted discomforts. The dissimilarities between such irritations and a true sense of hunger are quite sharp, the average person tied to the habit of eating at all hours of the day and night rarely permits himself to become hungry and consequently mistakes these morbid sensations for a valid call for food. As eating commonly relieves symptoms of distress, the individual becomes convinced that food was just the thing needed. Often it is a kind of eating binge; the individual eats to cover up psychological miseries, as the drunkard drinks to drown his.

True hunger is selective rather than indiscriminate; it does not gulp greedily, but frequently demands a specific type of food. On the other hand it does not demand "luxurious dishes" as appetite tends to do, but is satisfied with plain fare. The compulsive eater who is not genuinely hungry is often plagued with vague longings to eat, without knowing exactly what he wants to eat. Usually, he wants something highly *stimulating* to his taste buds, well seasoned, exotic.

Hunger is intermittent and manifests when there is a need for food. It is never continuous; individuals who are "always hungry" are really displaying pathological symptoms. Am I implying that most people do not really know when they are hungry? I am indeed. Beginning almost with birth and the three-times-a-day stuffing program that is common to our so-called modern civilization, average individuals in average communities never experience genuine hunger.

Since hunger is the normal indication of a need for food, it may be taken for granted that when hunger is lacking, no such immediate need exists.

Either the need is not present or the actual ability to make use of raw materials is absent. In the absence of hunger, there is no natural or normal reason why food should be taken. There are ample grounds for believing that the digestive system is in the best state to receive and digest food when real hunger is present, and that when hunger is absent the digestive processes are slowed or suspended. We have cultivated the habit of eating by the clock to such a point that we often persist in ignoring even a strong repugnance to food. Hungry or not, we eat as a matter of routine, as social activity, because we have nothing else to do, or because eating seems to relieve some of our worries.

The most important rule in our eating habits, and indeed in our daily lives, is this: *Never force food into the stomach either in health or in sickness, unless there is a definite demand for it as manifested by genuine hunger.*

In adults, alcohol, tobacco, coffee, a protracted sexual episode, strong emotions and enervation all result in a loss of the normal desire for food. Pain, fever and inflammation cause one to lose his desire to eat, as does abdominal distress. There is no better way for an adult to meet this situation than to refrain from eating until there is a return of hunger—until the breath is sweet, the tongue is clean, and there is keen relish for food. Food should be taken only when there is comfort and poise.

In acute disease, hunger is not present for the simple reason that the energies of the organism have been diverted into other channels. There is no energy to spare to carry on work like digestion, that can temporarily be dispensed with. Not only is nervous energy diverted to the task at hand, but there also is diversion of the blood to parts requiring extra blood for the unusual action. Digestion is suspended in such a mighty effort, just as it is when one engages in strenuous physical effort, such as running.

Yet food is often taken at such times under the medical dictum that we must eat to keep our strength. In such instances the food is sometimes thrown up, or may be rushed out of the digestive tract by means of a diarrhea. If not expelled in these ways, it becomes a burden in the digestive tract, further adding to the poisoning of the body.

Even where the unusable food materials may be expelled from the body, the effort of the body to get rid of the unwanted nourishment lessens the efficiency of the body's defensive and expulsive efforts in progress against the cause of the disease. Forces are diverted from the work of healing and wastefully expended in an effort that could be avoided by the simple expedient of fasting. This partial and temporary suspension of the remedial effort slows up the recovery of the patient. Indeed, the repugnance to food that is present may rightly be regarded as a "closed-for-repairs" sign placed at the entrance of the digestive tract. It should be heeded.

Sometimes we *think* we want food when we are sick, but this is a false desire that, if satisfied, increases our suffering. I recall a personal experience as a teenager. I suffered with a slight fever, malaise, foul breath, a bad taste in my mouth and general discomfort. In obedience to my inclination under the condition I went to bed. But I was hungry or thought I was. I thought I wanted sardines. I wanted them so badly I could almost taste them. I demanded sardines. My mother didn't think sardines would be advisable for a sick boy, but like other youngsters I had learned that if I protested long enough, my parents would "give in" even against their better judgment. I continued to demand sardines.

Finally my mother sent to a nearby store and purchased a can of sardines. She arranged them on a dish and brought them to my bedside. I took one small taste and gave the dish back to my mother. I found that I did not really want anything. My body wanted no food. Even though I knew nothing of fasting in those days, I instinctively fasted and was soon well without taking any drugs.

I have seen parents employ many means of coercion and persuasion in their endeavors to get sick infants and children to eat in spite of their refusal. A common mode of persuasion with children is to bribe them with promises of toys, candies or baseball mitts. "Eat this for mother," runs the common plea.

"The doctor wants you to eat this."

"If you do not eat you can't get well."

It is only ignorance that permits us to browbeat sick children with such false "truisms." In chronic illness the individual may believe he is hungry but his sensations are, in fact, nothing more than irritations of the digestive tract. These morbid symptoms end when the individual fasts. If the desire to eat was real indication of the need for food, the symptom pangs would increase as the fast progressed. The fact that the "hunger" ceases and the patient becomes comfortable is a sure indication that they have no relation to genuine hunger.

The statement sometimes heard that hunger ceases on the third day of the fast implies that true hunger is present during the first two days of the fast. This is usually not true. It is gastric irritation that ceases on the second, third or fourth day of the fast.

5

Four Reasons for Fasting

The purposes of fasting are many and varied; they range from bodily health factors and weight reduction to religious concepts and rituals—though the latter are usually for too brief a time to be considered as serious fasting, generally lasting no longer than a day at most.

Weight reduction is certainly a desirable goal, but should it be our only goal? Are there not other health factors involved in losing weight? Should there not be other clear cut physical and health benefits obtainable through a worthwhile fast?

Dr. Robert Walter, prominent for his work in *Hygiene*, was head of the world-famous *Hygienic* Walter's Park Sanatorium at Wernersville, Pennsylvania. He states that a moderate "hunger cure"—as fasting had been termed early German Nature Curists and early *Hygienists*—is exceedingly beneficial in a great number of diseases. In understanding the way fasting can help the human organism let us examine briefly here fundamental areas where total fasting, with the sole exception of drinking water, can play an important role. We have already begun to explore what we may call area number one—weight reduction. There can be no question that fasting produces the quickest, safest and most effective avenue available for weight reduction.

But it is important to note that in the cases of overweight individuals, weight reduction is an added benefit even when not the sole, or even the main reason for the fast.

A second reason is what I call physiological compensation, in which the delicate automatic balances of nature come into play. To expend on one side, nature must conserve on the other. This time-tested fact applies to all of the operations of living things, including human beings. If you have the water running in your bath tub and somebody turns on the water in the kitchen sink, the rate of the flow into the bath tub is immediately diminished. When the water in the kitchen is cut off, the rate of flow into the bath tub is immediately increased.

A similar phenomenon is witnessed in the operation of the body. If food is to be digested, much blood must flow to the digestive organs and we tend to become sluggish, even to fall asleep. If we force ourselves to do hard work, the process of digestion is practically suspended.

Fasting by conserving the energies of the body that are regularly employed in the work of the digestive system, permits the diversion of these energies to other channels with which to accomplish other work. Energy saved in one department may be expended in another.

A third reason is to secure physiological rest. This is rest of the digestive, glandular, circulatory, respiratory and nervous systems. In a general sense, the more food one eats, the more work must be performed by the organs making up these systems; when there is a great reduction in the amount of food taken, these ogans rest. When no food is taken at all, they rest most of all. It is not difficult to understand that when no food is eaten, the glands of the mouth and stomach, the whole digestive tube, the liver and the pancreas rest; it should be equally as easily understood that the heart and arteries are also relieved of a burden and secure rest. The glands of the body, other than those that secrete digestive juices, are also permitted to reduce their secretory activities. Respiration is slowed down and the nervous system has less work to do. All of this means rest.

There is a theory that the metabolism and inactivation of the fasting man resemble that of the hibernating animal. It says that only during the prenatal phase of man's existence is there greater immobilization of the digestive tract and muscles than during a fast. There is much truth in this theory, but we should recognize that the fasting man is not dormant, as is the hibernating animal, and is not as inactive as is the embryo. Indeed, so far as mind and muscles are concerned the faster, unless he goes to bed, relaxes his body and poises his mind, may be very active. It is true, however, that the more closely the faster can approach the inactivity of the prenatal stage of existence, the more rapid will be his progress. The rejuvenation of the cellular structures will be in keeping with his inactivity.

The fourth reason is the all important matter of elimination. J.H. Tilden, M.D., who was founder of the famous Dr. Tilden's Health School in Denver, Colorado, and edited and published two magazines and wrote several books, said: "After fifty-five years of sojourning in the wilderness of medical therapeutics, I am forced to declare, without fear of successful contradiction, that fasting is the only reliable, specific, therapeutic eliminant known to man."

Felix L. Oswald, M.D. agrees with him, saying: "Fasting is the great system renovator. Three fast-days a year will purify the blood and eradicate the poison-diathesis more effectively than a hundred bottles of expurgative bitters."

Nothing known to man equals the fast as a means of increasing the elimination of waste from the blood and tissues. Only a brief period elapses after food is withheld until the organs of elimination increase their activities and a real physiological house-cleaning is instituted.

As the fast progresses pent-up secretions or, more properly, retained waste, are thrown out of the body and the system becomes purified. Relief of irritations occurs; the body becomes rested. In a vital sense the individual is "made over." Perhaps but a few days are required to free the blood and lymph of their toxic excess, but the fast goes deeper than this and occasions the excretion of toxins that have long been stored in the less vital tissues.

The nutritive stringency created by the fast causes the body to break down (by autolysis) all superfluous tissues and nutritional stores and to make use of these in sustaining the functioning tissues of the body. In this process, stored toxins are released into the circulation to be carried to the organs of excretion and eliminated.

Dr. Oswald declares: "With no digestive drudgery on hand, Nature employs the long-desired leisure for general house-cleaning purposes. The accumulations of superfluous tissues are overhauled and analyzed; the available component parts are turned over to the department of nutrition, the refuse to be thoroughly and permanently removed." Elimination of superfluities and encumbrances, neither of which can be achieved in a state of surfeit, is compatible with increasing powers and with processes of physiological and even biological readjustment during a fast.

Excretion is a fundamental function of life and it is as essential to the continued existence of the organism as nutrition. More than a hundred years ago, Sylvester Graham who wrote *Science of Human Life*, and who launched the world's first health crusade in 1831 (Graham flour and Graham bread are named after him) pointed out that in all living bodies there is an economy of disassimilation and excretion co-equal with that of nutrition. So long as an organism is alive, assimilation and growth on one side, and excretion on the other are in constant operation.

There is a constant effort to maintain normal purity of the fluids of the body by unceasing excretion of waste and by expelling all non-usable substances that may be introduced. Anything that the body cannot utilize as food must be expelled, hence excretion must go on as continuously as the processes of nutrition.

Day and night, asleep or awake, from before birth to death, the processes that expel waste and toxins from the body never cease. To a great extent the two processes of nutrition and excretion are performed by different organs, although there is some overlapping. The energies of the organism are at all times divided between assimilation and elimination, but there are times when one process takes precedence over the other. In certain conditions of the body, excretion is much more important and assimilation is reduced to a minimum.

There is a theory that excretion is suppressed when food is taken. It is held that the body cannot assimilate and eliminate at the same time. While there is an element of truth in their theory, it is not strictly accurate.

Excretion must go on, even while food is being digested, else waste would accumulate and result in death from self-poisoning. It is safer to suspend the nutritive processes for a brief time than to suspend those of excretion, although a complete suspension of the nutritive processes would also be fatal. Only in a very limited sense is it true that "assimilation arrests elimination."

There is also a theory that the increased elimination that occurs during a fast is only incidental to the effort of the body to secure nutriment for its functioning tissues. Here the idea is that as the body liquidates its non-essential and least essential tissues, and uses these as nutrients with which to sustain the essential tissues, stored up toxins are released into the blood and lymph, and are carried to the organs of excretion and cast out. The search for nutrients is conceived to be primary while the excretion of toxins that results is secondary to this effort to find food.

I believe this concept holds much truth. Waste and toxins are stored in the tissues, especially in the fatty and connective tissues, and, as these tissues are liquidated, the stored toxins are released. This seems to be the reason for the long-continued increase of excretion, for it would seem that the toxic load carried by the blood and lymph would be eliminated in a few days by the immediate increase in excretion brought on by abstinence.

Yet is it rational to assert that a function as fundamental to living existence as that of excretion is secondary to any other body function? It is to be doubted. The energy of the two processes bears a more or less constant relation to each other. As fasting reduces energy expenditure in digestion, the sum of energy thus saved is available for use through other channels to carry out more efficiently processes and functions which become for the moment, more important than digestive action. The body is enabled to mobilize its forces for other purposes, such as elimination and healing.

That this is the correct interpretation of the action that occurs is shown both by the fact that rest without fasting will increase elimination, even if not to the same extent, and that a reduction of food intake also increases elimination. It appears that whatever lessens the work of the organism permits an increase in the work of elimination.

The actual increase in elimination in fasting is seen even before any demand is made upon the food reserves. It is especially noticeable in the increased output of the kidneys that have been previously depressed in function, as is often seen in heart disease. The increase in excretion is seen in these cases, even before there has been any increase in heart efficiency. There is also the fact that in the early part of the fast, as well as in its later stages, increase in elimination is out of all proportion to the amount of tissue liquidated. Increased energy for elimination seems to be at least partially responsible for the increase in this function.

There are those who ask: "Can fasting cure a cancer?"

My answer is that while I have seen cancerous growths greatly reduced in size during a fast, I have never seen one eliminated completely.

It has been observed that diseased tissues in the organism are the first to be broken down and salvaged by the body during the fast as it strives to meet nutritive requirements of vital and functioning tissues. Dr. Berg claims that this is the most important healing effect of the fast, an opinion with which I cannot wholly concur; the breaking down of such tissues does not represent more than a small part of the beneficial effect of the fast.

Dr. Berg, however, states of fasting in its relationship to tissues, and particularly to cancer:

"One assumes, perhaps too hastily, that it would be the diseased, altered tissues with their diminished power of resistance which would be the first affected by this. This is certainly not always the case, especially in cancer. One has often been able to determine that although the patient becomes thin, the tumor continues to grow; really a perfectly clear thing since the cancerous tumor is an autonomy and is most often encapsulated and not in any direct contact with the rest of the body."

While the concept of the autonomy of cancerous growths can be over-worked, it is true that in some cases, they do persist in growing even through a long fast. In other cases the cancerous growth is greatly reduced in size, although I have never seen one totally obliterated by fasting. *Benign tumors* on the other hand are frequently completely broken down and absorbed.

Berg adds: "Furthermore, through the fast, when no new foods are supplied, one desires to provide the body with the possibility of mobilizing all of its deposited waste products and oxidize and eliminate them." As the accumulated waste is largely already oxidized material, it is elimination rather than oxidation that is secured by the breaking down of tissues taking place during the fast. The excretion of dropsical effusions, edematous accumulations, swellings, infiltrations, and growths of various kinds is often rapid during a fast.

"I don't feel any different now than when I started my fast. I really feel fine."

The young lady who told me this had been without food for three days in the opening stages of a fast to lose weight. She had observed no change in her strength. Indeed, she experienced an exhilaration, a lightness almost euphoric in effect.

This is not an unusual experience. A fact that has been observed in thousands of instances is that great numbers of invalids, instead of losing strength while fasting, gain it. Invalids who were growing weaker on the many and varied "nourishing diets" that are commonly advised, will frequently begin to grow stronger as soon as they begin to fast. Paradoxical as it may appear, the weakest persons often derive the greatest benefit from a period of abstinence. Weakness, in most cases, is not due to lack of food, but to a toxic state of the body.

The popular idea runs that the weak must be "built up." They are told they are "too weak to fast." Even when the patient is growing steadily weaker while eating what is called "plenty of good nourishing food," it is assumed that the food build-up must go on. Never was there a greater error.

When a patient is so weak that he is unable to turn in bed, possibly in severe pain, and with fever, there is no power to digest food. Will the patient recover if fed like a harvest hand? Often he will, but the feeding will be no part of his recovery. If he dies, over-feeding at a critical time could have been a direct cause of his death. Will he recover, if he fasts? Not always. But he will be more likely to do so than if fed.

It is a popular idea that man is immediately and utterly dependent upon food supplies every few hours, and that he will grow weak and die if he misses a few meals. Well or sick, we are expected to eat three or more times each day. We are to be deaf, blind and silent to every signal of distress and eat in spite of such signals. If there is no desire for food, eat anyway; if there is actual repugnance for food, disregard it; if there is nausea, eat; if the digestive function is badly impaired or has been suspended, so that digestion is impossible, eat anyway. Such is the popular misconception.

How often do we read that some notable patient is now "able to take nourishment" only to have the next report state that the patient is worse? This is such a common occurrence that it is difficult to understand why the connection between the ill-advised feeding and the subsequent deterioration of the patient's condition is not quickly discerned. One notable example out of the past is the case of the world-famed actor, Joseph Jefferson, during whose last illness, Dr. Charles E. Page made the following memorandum from the published accounts of his illness:

"April 16th: Has not retained nourishment.

April 20th: The patient is better.

April 20th: Retained nourishment.

April 21st: More restless: condition less favorable."

Mr. Jefferson had pneumonia, a disease in which it is especially important not to eat. Further he had suffered with gastritis for several months before developing the pneumonia. His illness was at first described as an "attack of indigestion from an indiscretion in diet on a visit to a friend." During the pneumonia, he had no desire for food, and there was no possibility of digesting and assimilating it, but he was fed in spite of these circumstances. Forced feeding, alcohol and heart *stimulants* followed. After his death, it was announced that "his age was against him."

Thousands are thus yearly fed into premature graves. Today, as then, do we not read or hear of such cases. It is part of a process that goes on because the world still believes it can eat itself well.

Apparently it is difficult for us to learn anything from such experiences, although they occur daily. Due to the obscurity of most such patients, they do not make headlines. Going without food in these cases not only relieves pain, but it rests the heart and relieves the kidneys. Giving digitalis to *strengthen* the heart and morphine to *relieve* the pains and discomforts that follow injudicious feeding, instead of omitting food, may kill the patient. The sick man rallies when food is omitted and he relapses when feeding is prematurely resumed. These definite results should reveal the evil of feeding the acutely sick.

It is almost the invariable rule that the seriously acute sufferer gains strength as his symptoms decline through fasting until, by the time there is a natural call for food, his strength is often amazing. It is not rare that we see a patient who has been eating regularly but is too weak to get out of bed, gain strength almost from the beginning of a fast, until, by the end of a week or ten days of fasting, he is able to be up and walking around. I have seen patients so weak they would crawl up the steps while eating, and I have seen these same patients run up the same steps after a few days of fasting.

During the closing years of the last century and the early years of this, many fasters seem to have tried to ascertain how much work they could get out of their body while abstaining from food. They were proud of winning foot races, setting world's records in weight lifting, working longer hours and doing more work, both mental and physical, while fasting than while eating. Some of them kept late hours. Tanner ran a race with a reporter; Gilman Low set several world's records in lifting; Macfadden lifted weights while fasting; many continued their daily activities during prolonged fasts.

I know of one individual who worked in an office at detailed account analysis. He reported that his mind was keener and his mental reactions appeared to him to be not only sharper but quicker during fasting periods.

One faster was questioned by a newspaper reporter who refused to believe that the man he was interviewing, who had been on a fast for several days, did not suffer from physical weakness.

"I'll prove it," the faster told the reporter. "I'm fitter now than you are."

The reporter asked him if this were a challenge.

"Yes. I'll race you a hundred yards."

The race was arranged promptly, the faster and the reporter lined up, ran the course. The reporter was much younger than the faster, and much more the athletic type. But he lost to the man who hadn't had a mouthful to eat for days.

Another man, who had vast experience in the fast, had this to say to me: "The brain becomes wonderfully clear; the body grows into a recognition of its own power; languor, disinclination to mental and physical work disappears, and one enters upon his daily duties with a vim and energy and a delight that betokens the possession of the perfect and abounding health which is every man's birthright."

Of course the faster must at all times heed the instructions of the supervisor guiding the fast. This is above all true with physically weak individuals whose reserve strength may be below that of the average normal healthy person. In all cases, when the fast supervisor instructs that the fast be broken, this order must be heeded immediately.

There are cases in which the fast is broken only after two or three days. Fine. If this is what the expert orders—break it.

As in all other human activities, wisdom, caution and common sense must guide our actions. But in most cases the fast, under proper guidance, continued for the proper duration in relation to the individual physical needs and requirements, will leave the faster stronger rather than weaker in his general physical and mental capabilities and responses.

To take up every misconception in the public mind about fasting would require a special volume. But certain fallacies ought to be examined—and cleared away. The most important of these is the erroneous statement that fasting can kill.

Let us be very clear on one basic fact: to fast is not to starve. To starve is to abstain from food beyond the period when the fast must end; when the individual has reached a point at which weakness rather than strength sets in, or gives indications of setting in. Since the fast should and indeed must be conducted under expert professional direction, the director orders the fast broken before it ceases to be fasting and becomes starvation instead.

Can starvation kill if abstention from eating continues deep into the second or starvation stage of abstention?

It can; and in some rare cases it has, where common sense has been deliberately ignored.

Mrs. Gloria Lee Byrd, author of two books on outer space, died at the age of thirty-seven as a result of prolonged abstinence from food. She abstained from eating for sixty-six days. She had been instructed to fast for peace, she said, by 'J.W.' a ruler of outer space, who had called her from Jupiter. She was to continue her fast until 'J.W.' sent what Mrs. Byrd described as a 'light elevator' to Earth to take her to Jupiter.

It is not certain that she totally abstained from food for the whole of the sixty-six days. Physicians at the Washington, D.C. hospital where she died expressed the opinion that she had taken juices part of the time, but had been on a 'complete' fast during the last month of her life.

Here again we have an example of the misuse of terms. The news account states that she 'starved' herself for sixty-six days and then tells us that she was on a 'complete' fast for at least thirty days of her period of abstinence. As her fast was voluntary, even though undertaken under the belief that she had been instructed to do so by some being from outer space, she may be said to have fasted (in the true sense of this term) for a certain period without food, and to have begun to starve sometime in the latter part of this time. It may be that she died of starvation; it cannot be said that she died of fasting.

As the published account of her death provides us with no details of her size, the state of her flesh, her rate of loss, her activities while abstaining from food, and other details that should be in our possession in order to determine how long she fasted and when she began to starve, we will hazard no guesses about these matters. I judge from her picture that she was a small woman; she does not seem to have been fat. She had been an airline hostess and since in this profession women are commonly chosen above a certain height, we may assume that she was not a short woman. Perhaps fifty days would have been somewhere near her limit as a faster, but this would have also depended on her physical and emotional activities.

Mrs. Byrd became unconscious only four days before her death and did not regain consciousness.

What was done to her in the way of treatment during these last four days in the hospital is not revealed. It is physiologically impossible to starve to death before the skeleton condition is reached, but death may occur at any time, fasting or eating, from other causes.

Fasting, as I have defined it in this book, does not cause death. Death from lack of food can occur only after the total exhaustion of the body's food reserves. It does not immediately occur then, as it is still possible to maintain the functions of the vitally essential organs by sacrificing the less essential organs.

But death may result from an advanced condition of cancer or heart disease or Bright's disease or some other condition of this nature while the fast is in progress. In such cases it is not correct to attribute death to the fast. Those patients die without fasting and it is reasonably certain that in most cases they would die sooner if eating.

An example of a death falsely attributed to fasting is that of a nine-year old boy in Albany, New York in September, 1932. The coroner called it death brought on by starvation. The news account did not state how long the boy had been without food, but it did state that he collapsed while attending school.

Now, no boy that is near death from starvation attends school. In an actual state of starvation the boy would have lacked the strength to walk. He would have been confined to bed for several days prior to death. The account also stated that the boy was "seized with convulsions." Convulsions never complicate starvation. Such stories while they tend to keep alive the myth that the sick must eat "plenty of good nourishing food to keep up strength," are fallacies.

When anyone dies while fasting, sensational newspapers are almost sure to herald the death as one due to starvation, without knowing the conditions of the faster or actual details of the case. Such stories play up the starvation angle, and the general public is likely to get a distorted picture of fasting from such sources. What would be the result if some newspaper published the details of every death that occurs in a large city hospital for a whole year, giving the name of the physician in attendance, the name of the hospital where the death occurred, the drugs or operations employed— and attributed each death to the drugs or the operation? Such a procedure might not convince the public that drugging is a monster evil, but it would certainly cause consternation among physicians.

There are certain to be some failures of fasting to achieve lasting recovery. This is especially true in those far advanced cases that have turned to fasting as a last resort. It cannot be claimed that fasting will enable every man, woman and child regardless of his condition and the stage of the sickness, to recover good health.

Its limitations are those of the body. Fasting is not a *cure*. Healing is a spontaneous biological process and only such healing as the body is capable of doing can occur whether the patient feasts or fasts. Hopeless cases that have already reached the stage of irreversibility will not recover when, as an eleventh hour measure, the patient turns to fasting for help.

The danger most often is not, in fact, that the patient will be starved, but rather that he will be stuffed to death. Where a disease is terminal and there is no hope of recovery, it seems to me cruel to stuff the patient with overfeeding that can only increase the suffering of the dying.

8

Does Fasting Cure?

If fasting in general does not weaken the faster in weight reduction and even tends to increase strength—does it benefit in disease?

One of the leading practitioners in the field of fasting, George S. Weger, M.D., who headed the Weger Health School, Redlands, California, and wrote *The Genesis and Control of Disease* says: "The writer is willing to side with the enlarging minority and believe in the efficacy of the fast. Facts will not down. Nothing is more gratifying, no work more inspiring, than actually to witness complete recovery during comparatively short periods of fasting in diseases such as chronic eczema, urticaria of years' standing, varicose ulcers, gastric and duodenal ulcers, asthma, arthritis, colitis, amoebic dysentery, endocarditis, sinusitis, bronchitis, neuritis, Bright's disease, acute and chronic appendicitis, tic douloureux, fistula, psoriasis, all kinds of digestive disorders—urinary and bilary calculi, pellagra, glaucoma, lump on the breast, epithelioma, migraine, acidosis, pupura hemorrhagica, epilepsy, paralysis agitans, Reynaud's disease, and even locomotor ataxia. . . .

"Many other derangements could be added to the list, which is not by any means exhaustive, neither does it represent single experiences. Conclusions are based upon actual group results. Many will say, 'Preposterous!' Many will say there is no such thing as a 'Cure-All'! Others may damn with faint praise. To all doubters we must say in all seriousness that fasting, and a diet properly selected and combined, are the nearest approach to a 'Cure-All' that is possible to conceive—profoundly simple and simply profound."

Dr. Weger did not believe that fasting is a *cure* for disease: indeed, along with Dr.Tilden, he did not believe in *cures*. I account for his use of the term in this instance only by assuming that a man brought up in the belief in *cures* having had it instilled into his mentality throughout his term in medical college and through years of medical practice, here falls into the habit of using the term in a generalized sense rather than in the precise meaning it has taken on in modern thinking.

The view of *Hygienists*, and both Dr. Tilden and Dr. Weger had abandoned the practice of regular medicine for a *Hygienic* practice, is that fasting is not a *cure* in the modern meaning of this much abused term. Fasting does not *cure* anything. A fast is a period of physiological rest. It does not do anything at all. It is, rather, a cessation of doing. The rest provides an opportunity for the body to do for itself what it cannot do under conditions of surfeit and full activity.

The term *cure* comes from the Latin *cura* which was the equivalent of our word care. But the meaning of words is constantly changing. The biologist, A. D. Darbishire, formerly with the University of Edinburgh, in analyzing the changing meaning of words in his *Introduction to Biology* says: "When the adjective curious detached itself from its parent substantive, cure meant care. Thus cure first meant the care of the healthy, then the successful treatment of the sick, and lastly the drug supposed to drive away the malady. We speak of and even believe in a cough cure."

Today the word cure is variously defined as a medicine effective in treating disease, as a successful treatment of a disease or wound, or again as a system of treating disease. When we say that there are no *cures*, we simply mean that there are no methods or systems of treatment that in themselves restore health, whether the treatment is directed to a wound or a so-called disease. This is to say that there is and can be no such thing as a "successful method of treating disease." There is no "course of treatment" that will restore health. We go further and assert that disease should not be treated; that it should not be *cured*, that there is no need for a *cure*.

The attempt to restore the sick to good health without correcting or removing the cause of diseases is too often what is understood by *cure*. To *cure* in this modern usage, is to give a drug or to perform a rite, mechanical, surgical, or psychological, that will, it is hoped, restore health in spite of the continued operation of the cause of sickness.

The search for *cures* which is continuous is a search for means of restoring the sick to health by the application or administration of a treatment without the necessity of removing the cause or causes that are maintaining the impairment of health. As a recent example, cortisone was employed to *cure* arthritis, the cause of which is admittedly unknown. The cortisone was not supposed to remove the unknown cause. Cause was ignored and cortisone was administered. The first clearing up of symptoms was heralded with enthusiasm as a successful *cure*. But a short time elapsed before it was realized that this *cure* was as illusory as other *cures*.

The production of effects can be ended permanently only by removing the causes responsible for them. We behave as though we believe that effects can be erased and their production ended without the necessity of removing the causes producing them—that we can sober up a drunk man while he continues to drink, that we can prevent the evolution of cancer of the lungs while the man continues to smoke.

It is necessary that we learn the simple but fundamental lesson that when cause is removed the body can begin to heal itself. Removing cause does not do the healing; it only makes it possible for the restorative processes of the organism to perfect their work.

Healing, as distinct from *curing* is a biological process; it is not an art. A surgeon may bring the severed edges of a wound together and suture them, he cannot heal the wound. He may bring the ends of broken bones together and fix them so that they do not again become separated. But he cannot unite the two sections of the bone. The actual knitting of the bone is a process of life that only the living organism knows how to carry out. Man can neither duplicate nor imitate the process.

Briefly describing the processes by which the body repairs its injuries, Dr. Robert R. Gross of Hyde Park, New York, says: "We know precisely how a callus is formed to knit broken ends of a bone and the parts played by bone cells (*osteocytes*), the bone-forming membrane (*periosteum*), the *fibroblasts* (cell-producing fibrous tissues) and capillary blood vessels. We know a severed continuity of the skin heals by various so-called 'intentions' —first and second—by the appearance of fibroblasts and endothelial buds (embryological blood vessels) to form granulation tissue connecting the split skin layers and placing them in apposition to one another."

This somewhat technical description of some of the processes of healing a wound or broken bone actually bears out the truth that the remarkable process of healing as carried on by the living organism, employs the same processes in the production of new tissues, whether soft or bone tissue, that are employed in the production of skin, muscles, blood vessels, nerves, bones—the total organism—from conception.

Healing is accomplished by the same processes by which the tissues were first produced. I repeat: the production of new tissue (*histogenesis*) in healing a wound or knitting a broken bone, is the same as the process of producing new tissue in the original evolution of the organism from fertilized ovum to fully formed organism. These processes can neither be duplicated nor imitated by any disease-treater, whatever his medical bag of tricks may hold.

The secrets of healing are locked up in the living organism and there is nothing outside the organism that can usurp its prerogative of self-healing. We may study the processes by which healing is accomplished, but we cannot reproduce them. There may be a science of healing, but no art of healing, because art as such, is distinctive from the life processes. We are dealing not with the art of the physicians but with the work of living tissues.

Admitting that there are many circumstances, chiefly wounds, and traumatic conditions, in which a skilled surgeon can be of inestimable service, it remains tragically true that too often the "healing art" consists of throwing monkey wrenches into the vital machinery.

Once we have fully grasped the significance of the fact that healing is a process of life, that the processes by which healing is accomplished are as much a function of the living organism as the processes of digestion, respiration, circulation, elimination, reproduction, we can understand that so-called *cures* may come and go, but healing goes on endlessly. We will understand why almost anything may appear to *cure*, although there are no *cures*.

This brief description of the healing processes should underscore the fact that all healing is self-healing, and that fasting is therefore not a *cure*, in the sense that this word is now defined. When we say that fasting does not *cure* disease, we mean that it heals no wounds, knits no broken bones, it repairs no tissues, eliminates no poisons; it does none of the things that are parts of the processes of healing.

It does not initiate these healing processes, nor does it keep them in operation. The healing processes are spontaneous and ever-imminent, springing into activity the instant there is need for them.

There is a very radical sense, however, in which it may be said that fasting is an integral and essential part of the over-all process of healing: it is a part of the *remedial process* that is called disease—at least in many circumstances and conditions of life. When the body cuts off all desire for food and rejects it if eaten, it should be understood that the abstinence thus enforced is part of the over-all process by which health is restored.

As a physiological rest, fasting is merely one of the normal conditions for the efficient operation of the healing processes that are intrinsic to life. It provides opportunity for the body to do its own healing work in its own inimitable way and with less hindrance. When we place a sick person upon a fast, we do not do so with any idea that we are administering a *cure*, but with the idea that we are providing the organism with a much needed rest. Writers and lecturers who speak of the "fasting cure," or a "hunger cure" or of "therapeutic fasting" are simply victims of popular fallacies. They do not accurately describe the fast and its role in caring for the body.

Nor should fasting be called a rest *cure*, as it has been. Rest does not *cure*. The sick are no more *cured* by rest than are the well. Rest is one of the normal needs of life—as essential to continued existence as are food and air, warmth and sunshine, exercise and cleanliness. But it no more *cures* disease than does any of these other elements of nature's plan of hygiene.

Does fasting *cure*? Obviously, from the foregoing the answer is no. But it is also clear that fasting, used properly under correct supervision and guidance, can be a powerful silent ally in the body's healing process.

9

Fasting: Where and When?

Apart from our motivation and goals in fasting, the question of proper supervision, and other facets of fasting already considered, there are several basic considerations that should be discussed here: Where to fast, and when, and how long?

Although the questions appear simple on the surface, they present complex problems that cannot be answered as easily as one might imagine. For each is concerned with matters that relate to the individual, his personal physical condition and other factors of a variable nature.

The problem of when to fast for example, involves not only the matter of climatic conditions—which may become extremely important—but also the question of how quickly it may be considered essential for the individual to begin the fast.

Because fasting lowers one's resistance to cold and the faster is easily chilled, fasting is more pleasant generally in warm weather than in cold. For this reason, there are those who advocate fasting in summer. On the other hand, Dr. Oswald considered winter entirely suitable for fasting and pointed to the example of hibernating animals to support his view. Moreover, waiting for summer could involve procrastination during which the condition of the patient might deteriorate. Chronic disease tends to evolve into more serious stages with the passage of time.

I believe that a fast should be entered into at any time of the year it may be needed, without reference to the climate. No impairment of health should be risked awaiting changes in climate. If one stays indoors and keeps warm, it is as easy and safe to fast in winter as in summer. Fasting is equally as beneficial at one time of year as at another, and the logical rule should be: *Fast when there is a need for it.*

It is best, when uncomfortable in any way, to stop eating until feeling well, without respect to the time of year.

There are varying degrees of inability to appropriate food in the various states of impaired health, and in all of these, a period of abstinence will hasten recovery. One should not wait until one is suffering with serious disease before instituting remedial measures. Take care of the small illnesses at the right time and in the right way and the more serious illnesses will not evolve. It is unfortunately true, as Dr. Charles E. Page, who lived in Melrose, Mass. and was an outstanding *Hygienist*, says, that "nearly all patients continue eating regularly, until food becomes actually disagreeable, even loathsome, often; and after this, every effort is exhausted to produce some toothsome compound to tempt the appetite. Furthermore, and often worst of all, after the entire failure of this program, the patient can, and usually does, take some gruel or some sort of 'extract' which he can drink by holding his breath. All this tends to aggravate the acute symptoms, and to fasten the disease in the chronic form upon the rheumatic patient, or to insure rheumatic fever; and the same principle holds in nearly all acute disorders, it is well to remember."

Fasting is a preventive program in that it initiates the cleansing process before serious developments have occurred. Fasting is used successfully in many cases of serious chronic illnesses—in advanced stages—and this will be explained later. But certainly it is wise to "nip in the bud" all such developments rather than to wait until the trouble has become formidable before doing anything about it. A great number of those who are reading this book are already in advanced stages of disease and they will desire to know what they can expect from a judicious fast. Much of this book will be devoted to answering such questions for them. At this point, it is only essential that I say that, while fasting can save many lives it is too much to expect it to save all lives without respect to the condition of the patient at the time the fast is undergone.

Dr. Page also says: "There is neither pleasure nor nourishment in forced feeding, only pain, poisoning and starving. The fasting cure universally and rationally applied, would save thousands of lives every year."

Dr. Page further urges the immediate launching of a fast wherever indicated, emphasizing that in serious cases, "plenty of good food" as the saying goes, can kill far more quickly than it can benefit.

The question, when to fast, is answered: When the need arises, as quickly as can be arranged, under advice, and without great expectations of immediate miraculous developments, instant recovery, or overnight slenderizing to sylph-like proportions.

We have been brought up in the belief that we can recover health in one swallow of a pill. That weight which has taken years to amass will vanish in a matter of hours. In cases of serious disease, the same lack of realism is seen. The layman is unacquainted with the state of deterioration in organs and tissues, and is likely to expect, even demand, results that are impossible. A man who has taken forty or fifty years to evolve the diseased state that he presents when he undergoes a fast, may expect to get well in a few days or a few weeks.

The sooner we can divest our minds of this false notion, the better will we be able to comprehend the fact that getting well, which is an evolution in reverse, requires time and persistence. One fast is often not enough. The chronic sufferer, after long years, will have not only to persist in his efforts to undo the effects of a life-time of wrong living, but he will have to exercise patience in his efforts.

Yet there are also conditions in which a fast, at least of any length, is inadvisable, even impossible. In states of great emaciation, in advanced stages of heart disease, cancer, diabetes, and in advanced tuberculosis, there is nothing to be gained from a fast. Fasting in cancer of the liver and in cancer of the pancreas is especially to be avoided. Where there is great fear of the fast, it is well not to undertake it.

In pregnancy, fasting should be resorted to only in cases of urgent necessity. In cases of morning sickness, common in the early stages of pregnancy, fasting a few days will prove of benefit. Apart from this, if there is no acute disease that makes a fast essential, the woman should avoid fasting while pregnant. By this I do not, of course, mean that she cannot miss an occasional meal or even fast for a day or so, if she finds it helpful.

As fasting causes the milk of the nursing mother to diminish, and it is not increased when feeding is resumed, the nursing mother should avoid fasting unless her adviser considers it an urgent necessity. It is important for the expectant mother to maintain high-level health during pregnancy and the nursing period.

A student of *Hygienics* once made the following half-joking comment: "The trouble with fasting is, there's no place to do it in."

The environment of the faster is too often filled with difficulties and obstacles. Home should be an ideal place, but usually isn't. This is partly because of the wide-spread ignorance about fasting. Also, the home too often is located amid the noise and fumes of the city, where the water is "drugged" until it is almost unfit to drink. With a little effort it is possible for the man in the city to obtain pure water, but pure air is not possible.

Perhaps the greatest obstacle to fasting at home is the almost inevitable opposition of the faster's family and relatives, not to mention his neighbors and friends. They will not let him alone. They plead with him and badger him to eat. They tell him he is crazy, that he will kill himself, that he is looking bad, that if he does not cause his own death, he is sure to do serious harm to himself.

They may become angry, even hysterical, in their efforts. They quarrel with him and annoy him so much that fasting is all but impossible. They call in a physician to persuade him to break the fast. They may even call in the police or threaten commitment in a mental institution.

Tasty tidbits are prepared for the purpose of tempting him. They can turn the fast into a grotesque nightmare. I have had to take patients out of their homes and send them elsewhere to complete the fast.

On the other hand, where there is family cooperation, a fast in the home is carried out with ease, peace and success.

It should be carried on amid quiet, peaceful surroundings, where the air is pure, the water fresh and uncontaminated, and the people congenial. As it should also be properly supervised by one experienced in conducting fasts, the best place for fasting is an institution in which fasting is regularly carried out.

A *Hygienic* institution located in the country and headed by an experienced supervisor, forms an ideal combination for a fast. Fasting is not merely refraining from eating for a required period. It involves rest, sunbaths, bathing, quiet, peace, and the care of the patient through the period of recuperation after the fast is broken. All of this requires knowledge and experience.

For most people, fasting is an unusual experience. This is particularly so if it is a first fast. The faster is likely to experience unfounded anxiety, uncertainty, mental perturbation, even fear. In addition he experiences new feelings and sensations that may disturb him. For these reasons alone, the best place to fast is at an institution, under the guidance of a man of wide experience in fasting.

How long should one fast? What is the time schedule? There are several different views about this and much discussion has been engaged in over these issues. Ideally, the answer is basically that the fast should continue until the return of hunger. Practically, however, this is not always possible, and it is rarely wise in any event to set an arbitrary limit to the duration of the fast.

No man is wise enough to predetermine the amount of fasting that will be required in a given state of the organism, nor can one tell in advance how much fasting will be safe in a particular case. The experienced man does not launch a fast with the idea that the patient is going to break any fasting records.

Fasting is not a stunt, nor a contest. The supervisor starts the patient on the fast with an objective in view—to reduce weight, to lower blood pressure, to relieve the body of accumulated waste, to rest a tired nervous system, to bring about rejuvenation of the individual, or whatever may be the specific goal. He carefully watches the faster and the day-by-day developments and breaks the fast when his object has been attained or before any danger to the faster has developed.

No living thing can go indefinitely without food, but fasting is always safe within the limits of the organism's power of self-help. As this limit is well demarcated, there is little likelihood that the experienced practitioner will mistake it and carry the fast beyond the point of safety. If the fast is continued, nature herself will always indicate when the fast should be broken.

Arbitrary limits are justified only if the patient has limited time in which to fast and be ready to return to work, or in those cases where a long fast is inadvisable. Other than these instances, the only satisfactory plan of conducting a fast is to be guided by the day-by-day developments in the physical state of the faster.

By this rule, a fast may last a few days, a few weeks or a few months. The longest fast I have ever personally conducted was one of ninety days. Two other patients passed seventy days, and many have gone beyond sixty days. Such long fasts are not the rule, nor can every faster safely continue so long. Each fast must be conducted according to the needs and the abilities of the individual.

The practitioner who arbitrarily sets a predetermined limit to the fast does not do justice to the faster. To set a limit of three days or a week or for twenty-one days, as some do, is to break the fast in the great majority of instances far in advance of the time it should be broken. Nor should the faster start out with the idea that he is going to try to set a record or to reach a certain goal in terms of number of days. The only logical rule is the following: *Let developments determine the length of the fast.*

In some cases a series of short fasts is preferable to one long fast. In general, one lengthy fast produces better results than a series of short ones. It is not always possible for a patient to take a series of short fasts. The time required is often too great and the expense prohibitive. And such a program, unless rigidly supervised, is capable of producing harm such as never results from a properly conducted long fast. There is the fact also that a program of alternating feeding and fasting tends to become more difficult for the individual to carry out.

Often the periods of abstinence are just long enough for the faster to become adjusted to the fasting process, then they are broken. Each time the patient fasts he is forced to go through the same experience. Never experiencing the comfortable stages of the fast, he tends to rebel against another fast, he hesitates, draws back, and dreads the whole routine.

In spite of the difficulties attending a series of short fasts, there are cases in which this is all that can be done, and then the plan should be undertaken with determination, but under supervision, to the end that the greatest good may be accomplished by it. These questions of where, when, and for how long are seen to be variables that must be handled and decided upon with common sense. The approach must be flexible, humane, understanding, wise. We are dealing with human beings, and not machines.

10

What to Expect while Fasting

Whether undertaken for reasons of weight reduction, or general health, or for some special physical impairment, the fast involves certain developments which should be examined and understood. These developments are for the most part mild, particularly where the individual is fasting only to reduce weight.

Let it be understood: I do not think it is possible to over-emphasize the fact that the physical sensations of fasting are, for the most part, far more pleasurable than the real or illusory delights of feasting. The patient, for example, who has previously suffered from being forced to eat when he had no desire for food, is likely to feel a great sense of relief and satisfaction from the outset of the fast.

Whatever the condition of the faster at the start, it is true that a fast can sometimes be somewhat uncomfortable, at least in certain of its stages. It is also true that in most cases the faster is more comfortable than when he was eating. Many can go through protracted fasting in a relaxed state with little or no discomfiture.

During the fast, every abnormal sensation, every discomfort, every ache and pain is likely to be blamed upon the fast. This may be true even though, as the fast proceeds, discomfort ceases. The condition of the individual's own tissues is the chief cause of the symptoms he experiences in the beginning. As these tissues are cleansed, discomforts disappear.

Most of us know something of the suffering and prostration brought on by the "withdrawal symptoms" of the inebriate when he is taken off alcohol. In a parallel way many who go on fasts have become so used to *food stimulants* through the years, that they go through a period of depression similar to that of the inebriate deprived of his alcohol. They may become nauseous and vomiting may occur. They may become irritable, sleepless, weak; there may be pains and aches in the body; there may be severe headache. It is not proper to call these developments "withdrawal symptoms," in my opinion. It is important to know that they are evanescent, of brief duration, are rarely severe.

Sometimes, to avoid and to ameliorate these symptoms, the faster is given fruits. I doubt that this is wise. With these foods, the fast is interrupted when the first signs of discomfort appear, and then it is resumed after two or three days of light eating of this nature.

The interruption with light feeding may have to be repeated two or three times during a fast of considerable length, if this plan is resorted to. It is doubtful that the interruption saves the faster a single slight twinge of discomfort and it is certain that it prolongs the time he has to be under observation. If the faster will grit his teeth, clench his fists, grin and bear the evanescent discomforts until the crisis is over the first time, there will be no recurrence of the symptoms. Frequently such a crisis is of extremely brief duration, no more than an hour or so. Only infrequently does it last longer than three to four days.

In addition to the foregoing general developments in fasting, there are a number of specific areas where changes and developments are usual and should be understood. Even though they present no problem or serious difficulty whatsoever, they should, as a part of the fasting routine, be discussed frankly with the experienced *Hygienist* who is directing the fast.

When one starts a fast, certain physical developments occur almost invariably and should not cause alarm. Chief among them are: The tongue coats heavily, a bad taste develops in the mouth and breath acquires a bad odor. Teeth may become pasty. The whole complex resembles the tongue, mouth and breath in fever. Indeed, there are fasting advocates who liken this to the depurative work of an acute illness, a *fever*.

Disagreeable as this condition may be, it represents a cleansing process. As the body unloads its toxic burden, a process of slow clearing of the tongue begins at the tip and on the sides and gradually clearing backward and towards the middle, until, by the time hunger returns, the tongue and mouth are clean and the breath sweet.

However light the urine may be at the beginning of the fast, it will become very dark and foul within a few hours to a day after the fast is started. It may become almost black in many cases and the odor will be very strong. After a week to two weeks, depending on the condition of the faster—the urine begins to clear, becomes lighter, loses its strong odor until by the time hunger returns it is normal in color and odor. The whole procedure is part of the evidence that the kidneys are engaged in throwing out unusual quantities of waste. Urine tests verify this fact. As purification continues, the urine returns to normal.

Loss of weight that results from fasting is consequent upon the utilization of the body's reserves in nourishing the vital tissues and the excretion of toxic accumulations. This loss should be regarded as part of the process of purification and the resulting improvement should be welcomed. The degree of unwholesomeness of the tissues helps to determine the rapidity with which weight is lost.

Loss is greatest in the early days of the fast, fat people losing at a faster rate than thin individuals. There are however, thin individuals who because of the toxic state of their tissues lose as rapidly as overweight fasters during the first few days. Losses at this stage range from a pound and a half a day, at the start of the fast, to four to six pounds in very stout individuals. After a few days of fasting, the rate of loss slackens. In the later stages of a long fast, less than a quarter of a pound a day may be lost.

It is easily possible to exaggerate the importance of weight loss in any consideration of fasting. The emaciated person who remains thin on his various "weight gaining" diets may be very reluctant to lose more weight, although generally after the fast, he will gain weight on much less food than he has been in the habit of eating. It is an error to think that fasting is of benefit only to fleshy people.

The *feeling* of weakness, sometimes experienced during a fast is due, in the main to functional inactivity. There is a general functional let-down as the organism takes full advantage of the proffered opportunity to rest. The heart slows, circulation slows, there is a slowing of respiration. The glands of the body reduce their activities. In general, the tired body heaves a sigh of relief and goes to bed. This is just what is needed and proof that it is beneficial is seen by the fact that vigor returns as the body rests and is cleansed, long before food is taken. Indeed weakness during the first few days of the fast may be nothing more significant than an absence of the accustomed *stimulation*.

Many people undertake to fast with the mistaken idea that the cleansing processes carried on during this period are necessarily of extremely trying and of disagreeable nature. This is true in only a minute percentage of cases; it is by no means the rule. On the contrary, most fasters go through even long fasts without the development of any dramatic or extraordinary crises. Most of the work of excretion is carried on without the production of troublesome crises. When a crisis does develop it should be welcomed, as it is almost always of a remedial nature.

Skin eruptions rarely develop during the fast, but are definitely eliminative processes when they do occur. Giddiness, fainting, palpitation of the heart, and symptoms of this nature, though not common, should not be regarded as crises. They present no danger to the faster.

Perhaps the most annoying development that occurs while a fast is in progress is that of nausea and vomiting. Not only is it a trying time while it lasts, but the faster is very weak also. Fortunately, there can be no doubt that this crisis is definitely beneficial and it does not occur in more than fifteen percent of cases. Nausea and vomiting can develop on the first day of the fast or at any time thereafter. Generally, a crisis develops after several days of abstinence. In a few instances they develop after four or more weeks of fasting.

What is ejected is usually a rather abnormal and watery bile with considerable mucus. The liver works over-time (for a day to a few days) and much of the bile thus turned out is regurgitated into the stomach, and is thrown out. The faster is so greatly benefited by the ordeal that he is well compensated for the discomfort. These episodes may last a day or they may last two, three, four days or a week. Rarely does vomiting persist beyond a week. The faster's strength returns when vomiting ceases.

If it persists for several days and water is not retained there is some inevitable dehydration. This is a serious matter, especially in cases where vomiting lasts for several days. The possibility of breaking the fast must be considered promptly. The faster is weakened by the dehydration and the recovery of strength is slow. If there is diarrhea along with the vomiting, and this occurs very rarely, the dehydration is more severe.

In such cases, if vomiting does not subside after a reasonable time, break the fast. This is not always easy as there is a tendency to vomit the food as well as the water. In supervising some fasters, I have often tried several kinds of juice before finding one that could be retained.

Diarrhea in a fast is not as common as vomiting, but it does occur occasionally. When it does develop, it may come at any period of the fast, even after thirty-five days. The discharge is composed of bile, mucus and retained feces. This crisis is undoubtedly of a cleansing character. It may be viewed in the same light as the diarrhea that accompanies marked edema in nephritis (Bright's disease) by which much of the edematous fluid is expelled from the body. That this ever occurs in non-fasters I am not sure, but it is a common development in fasting a dropsical case.

11

Nine Basic Steps

Let me warn emphatically that fasting is a much more complicated process than generally realized even by some of its ardent advocates. It involves much more than merely going without food. There is an art to fasting as well as a science of fasting. The uses of fasting seem, at times, almost unlimited. Its inconveniences are not great, its dangers are few and rarely seen. Yet for the most satisfactory results it must be conducted in accordance with a few well-ascertained rules and techniques by an experienced man. It is not a process to be left to the guidance of anyone of meager knowledge or no experience in conducting fasts.

Paradoxically, less supervision of the fast is required in acute disease than in chronic disease. When disease is the result of years of wrong life, and if the condition of the patient is one of grave weakness, with severe organic impairment, much skill will be required to take the individual through a fast of sufficient duration to accomplish the desired results.

In such situations, it would be hazardous to rely on inexperienced and untrained men. I am aware that there are some untrained laymen attempting to conduct fasts. I believe it is vitally important to investigate beforehand to be sure you have the best and most experienced man available. In this connection I must point out also that, while there are several schools of so-called healing recognized by law in this country, few of the practitioners of any of these schools have any knowledge of and experience with fasting. We cannot select any *doctor* at random, without knowing his special training, to supervise a fast.

It is a fundamental rule of *hygienic* practice that all the needs of normal physiology are present in states of illness. And in periods of abstinence, they must be met according to a degree of need and functional ability, to the end that organic and functional integrity may be preserved or restored. Let us understand this clearly: when we fast we do not also cease to breathe or to take water. There is never an absence of need for oxygen; we continue to become thirsty at intervals and we drink. Fasting is abstinence from food, not abstinence from all of the essentials of life. And it is abstinence from food only in the sense that we abstain from taking in the raw materials of nutrition for a period of time, while the body draws on its stored-up supplies. We still need and use food.

Fasting is not suspended animation. Indeed, although it is a period of greatly reduced activity, some of the processes of life are actually accelerated during periods of abstinence. The ordinary needs of life: food, air, water, warmth, sunshine, activity, rest, sleep, cleanliness, poise of mind, remain basic needs of the fasting organism.

Food (nutriment) with which to sustain the functioning tissues of the body is obtained from the reserve stores within the body. Water is taken according to the demands of thirst; warmth is required so that the body does not become chilled; sunshine is needed in keeping with the somewhat reduced metabolic activities of life; cleanliness is still a requirement; sleep is a necessity; mental and emotional stabilization is especially important.

This means that the techniques of fasting are significant and should at least, in a broad general sense, be recognized and understood by anyone interested in this field or contemplating a fast.

Where do these techniques begin? Some say they should begin long before the fast starts—with the earliest stages of fast preparation!

1. PREPARATION

Many complicated plans have been designed to prepare the individual or patient for a fast. Some of these involve a period on special foods intended to empty the intestinal tract of material before the fast is started. Others are rituals involving fasting a day, eating two days, fasting two days, eating four days, and so on in this manner, with the goal of gradually preparing one for a fast of considerable length. All such plans are wasteful of the patient's time and money, since they revolve around the idea of feeding at a time when a fast is needed. As there is no reason why one may not go into a fast abruptly and without these rituals, they are not recommended here. The truly essential preparation is in the mental and emotional attitudes.

If you can understand the wisdom and rationality of fasting, and rid your mind of all fear of this perfectly normal process, you can fast with ease. Satisfy yourself that the fast will prove to be highly beneficial and enter upon it without fear and anxiety. Mental unrest and fear can make fasting difficult or impossible in cases in which it would otherwise prove of the greatest possible benefit. When I first started my work, I served for a few months under the direction of Milo A. Crane, M.D., who conducted the Crane Sanitariums in Elmhurst, Illinois. Dr. Crane never placed a patient on a fast if the patient feared it. Instead, he would put him on a diet and permit him to mingle with the other patients. Usually within a few days the patient would ask if he could not fast.

This is one of the advantages of being with others. One sees and realizes that they are not starving but actually benefiting. Fears vanish before reality.

2. REST

The techniques of fasting are based on simple physiological principles. They do not involve the need for nor the use of any measures that are foreign to the regular needs of the living organism. Treatments, special modalities, and forcing measures have no place in fasting. The most important technique of the fast is that of reducing activity, mental, sensory, and physical, to a bare minimum, so that the energy of the faster may be conserved and his healing and excretory processes may be accelerated.

The faster should bear in mind the simple rule of compensation. *In order to expend on one side, nature must conserve on the other.* What he does not expend in unneeded activity is available for use in elimination and repair.

Physical rest is secured by ceasing physical activities, by resting in bed, by relaxing. Physical activities expend considerable energy and prevent the recuperation of energy that is essential to restoration of normal nerve energy.

Mental rest is secured by curtailing mental activities and emotional unrest. Debating highly controversial issues is harmful. Allowing oneself to become upset or involved in trivial disputes of any nature is harmful. Emotional poise is the secret of mental rest. It is not always easy for the faster to cease worrying or to overcome anxiety, but everything constructive should be done to provide for tranquility.

Sensory rest is secured by retiring to a quiet place and avoiding use of the eyes in reading, viewing television, going to the movies or similar eye-straining activities. Noise is especially destructive of poise and wasteful of energy. Quiet, peace, and sensory inactivity provide for conservation of energy.

In using rest, however, we do not urge a state of suspended animation nor dormancy, nor a state of embryonic passivity. What is sought here is the absence of strain, the physical sense of peace by which rest becomes possible.

Rest does not heal, but is one of the essentials of efficient healing, as well as in maintaining health. It is of great value to the enervated and toxemic. Not *tonics* and *stimulants*, not *sedation* and *tranquilization*, nor *hypnotization*, but rest is the great need of the organism that has been lashed into impotency by stimulation and excesses in food, sex, emotional unrest, work and the various deficiencies from which man suffers.

Organs that have been lashed into impotency by overwork and *stimulation* may be rested into full functioning vigor. Added *stimulation*, whatever its nature, only further depletes them.

3. ACTIVITY

The faster rests during the time he abstains from food for the reason that in the normal exercise of the functions of life, feeding and activity should balance each other. There are authorities who permit their fasters to take long walks and require them to take daily exercise of various kinds. In reducing fasts, some moderate exercise, under supervision is permissible. For other fasts I believe even moderate exercising is a needless expenditure of energy and a waste of reserves. Activity should be geared to the food eaten. When no food is taken, activities should be reduced to a minimum. Rest is the need, not expenditure.

4. WARMTH

A faster's resistance to cold is likely to be lower than that of the person who is eating regularly. He chills easily. Chilling inhibits elimination, increases the discomforts of the faster and causes a more rapid utilization of reserves. It is important, therefore, that the faster keep warm. This is necessary even in July and August. The feet, in particular, should be kept warm. Cold feet will prevent the faster from sleeping.

5. WATER

The faster will be thirsty at intervals, though rarely as often as when he was eating. The normal demand for water should be met with the purest water available. Mineral waters and waters with a bad taste are not advisable. A soft spring water, rain water, distilled water, filtered water or any water that is free of impurities is acceptable.

It should be taken only as thirst demands. There is nothing to be gained by drinking large quantities of water, despite a lack of demand for this, on the theory that this flushes the system. It is true that the more water one drinks the more fluid will the kidneys excrete, but this does not represent an increase of elimination of waste. Indeed it may result in a lessening of the amount of waste excreted.

In summer, there may be a desire to drink cold water. Cool water is excellent, but very cold or ice water may slow down and retard recovery. Hot water may be relished under certain conditions more than cold water or water at room temperature. In some cases hot water may be sipped in moderation with the advice or permission of the supervisor; in others its use is inadvisable.

6. BATHING

There is the same need for cleanliness while fasting as while eating. Bathing should be performed daily or as often as needed. The bath should be of a character to cause the least amount of energy expenditure. To insure this the following requirements should be observed.

(a.) The bath should be of short duration. The faster should not remain long under the shower or in the tub. The common practice of soaking for long periods in water is enervating and should be avoided.

(b.) Bath water should be lukewarm, neither hot nor cold. It requires considerable energy expenditure to resist both heat and cold. The closer the temperature of the bath water is to the temperature of the body, the less energy expenditure will be occasioned. Bear in mind, always, that bathing is for cleanliness and not for any alleged *therapeutic* effects. Bathe quickly and get out of the water.

(c.) If the faster is very weak and is unable to take his or her own bath, a sponge bath in bed may be given by an assistant.

7. SUNBATHING

Sunshine is an essential nutrient factor in both plant and animal nutrition and is helpful while fasting. It should not be thought of as a *cure*, for it is not, but as a normal element in the regular nutritional processes of life. Its role in calcium metabolism is especially important, but it is also important in phosphorus utilization and in assuring strength of the muscles. Indeed, it serves several important purposes in the normal processes of life and is of far greater importance to us than we generally realize.

Unless overdone, sunbathing results in relaxation and no measurable expenditure of energy. If the sun is too hot, if the bath is too prolonged, if getting to and from the solarium is too taxing on the patient, any of these factors may result in an excessive expenditure of energy. It is necessary to "temper the wind to the shorn lamb" in supervising the sunbathing. To accomplish this, the following rules should be observed:

Take the sunbath in the early morning while it is still cool, or in the late afternoon during the summer. In mild weather, when it is not hot at midday, a sunbath may be taken at any time of the day that the temperature is comfortable.

Start the sunbath with five minutes of exposure for the front of the body and five minutes for the back. On the second day this may be increased to six minutes on each side. Increase the exposure one minute a day for each side, to a maximum of thirty minutes for each surface. It will be well to level off at this exposure time.

If the fast is continued beyond twenty days, reduce the exposure to about eight minutes on front and eight minutes on the rear surfaces, and continue this exposure until after the fast is broken.

At any time if the sunbath leaves the faster weak or irritated, the duration of the exposure should be reduced. Avoid overdoing.

8. PURGES

It is sometimes claimed, completely erroneously in my opinion, that during the fast, it is necessary to keep the bowels, kidneys and skin active to carry away the toxins released into the circulation by the liquidation of tissue. Daily enemas or saline purges are advised to clean the bowels, much water drinking and even diuretics are advised to keep the kidneys active; sweat baths are employed to keep the skin active.

All of these forcing measures are not only unnecessary, they are actually hurtful. There is nothing that so safely and so certainly increases kidney action as the fast itself. The bowels empty themselves during a fast as often as there is a need for them to do so. If no need arises, they take a long-needed rest. The skin is not an eliminating organ and sweat baths are delusions. These measures further enervate the faster and tend to inhibit rather than accelerate elimination. These suggested techniques are harmful and should be avoided.

9. SUFFERING

It has been said that the fast should not be continued when the faster is suffering greatly, as in some general health impairment. The fact is that it is precisely under these circumstances that digestive and assimilative powers are lowest. The greater the suffering the less able is the sufferer to take and digest food. When the discomfort passes, the practitioner will know when to feed the patient.

Fasting tends to end suffering and the faster suffering may expect relief in a much shorter time if he continues to fast than if he breaks the fast.

12

Breaking the Fast

It is strange that the following simple truth, so obvious a truth indeed, is so difficult for many to grasp: the ideal moment to break the fast, of course, is at the time when hunger returns. As hunger returns, the tongue clears, the breath becomes sweet and there is a clean taste in the mouth. All the indications are that the body has completed the work of cleansing itself and is ready to resume eating.

There is usually a watering of the mouth and a strong desire for food. Does hunger always return? The correct answer is: nearly always. In terminal cases, such as advanced cancer, advanced tuberculosis, serious heart disease, and other conditions where death is merely a question of time, hunger rarely recurs. In all savable cases, and in those near normal individuals who fast, hunger never fails to put in its appearance at the right time.

Indeed it frequently recurs well in advance of the exhaustion of the body's reserves. This is particularly true following an acute disease. Within a day or two after all acute symptoms have subsided, in almost all such cases, the invalid will express a desire for food, although his body may still be amply supplied with reserves to carry him through many more days of abstinence.

With the exceptions noted, the fasting chronic sufferer can count on the same thing. Indeed, the difficulty he is likely to experience is not a failure of hunger to return, but in controlling himself and his appetite when it does.

After a fast of considerable length there is a period of several days, lasting up to two weeks, during which the individual feels hungry most of the time. If he will control his eating until this initial period of hunger has passed, he will settle down to a more normal appetite and the danger of overeating will pass.

Uncontrolled, he may eat so much during this period that he loses much that he gained in the fast. One important advantage of fasting in an institution is that control continues until the normal eating level is stabilized. In such an institution the health seeker's diet is carefully supervised;

he is not permitted to overeat. At home, he must be a more self-disciplined man than the average if he is to avoid overeating.

For numerous reasons most fasts are broken before the return of hunger. In a small percentage of cases, the faster is too thin or too weak to carry the fast to a natural termination. In many instances, there is a lack of time or funds, or there may be an unwillingness to fast so long.

Some fasters, even when fasting solely for health reasons, object to getting so thin. Most of them are anxious to end the fast as soon as they are free of their annoying symptoms. Many have the idea that they can complete the recovery begun with the fast by shifting to a diet. This is a mistaken notion, but it is not easy to convince those who are attracted to this half-way notion. They usually regret their action—afterward.

Some go on a fast during their vacation and have but a limited time for fasting, breaking the fast, and getting ready to return to work. Others feel that they can be away from their business or their family for only a certain period of time. There are a thousand personal reasons for ending the fast short of its natural termination. In many instances the results of these short fasts are disappointing. In some instances the premature breaking is the difference between complete success and partial failure.

A job only half done is not done at all. Certainly health is worth a little added effort. Missing a few more meals is a small price to pay for the results that can accrue to the individual willing to make the effort required.

The animal breaks his fast on whatever food is available at the time he resumes eating. On the whole, animals seem to be better controlled than man. They are not inclined to glut themselves when they break a fast, but may take but a small portion of food in doing so. A dog that has fasted for nearly a month, for example, may take but a few sips of milk at a time and may refuse all flesh for the first four to six days after he resumes eating. If man's instincts were still as reliable guides to eating as are those of the animals, I doubt that we would need to supervise the breaking of a fast.

It is possible to break a fast with any food available. Either whole fruits or whole vegetables may be used. In order not to overconsume food, we have found it advisable to weigh the food for the first few days.

Dr. Virginia Vetrano, who has been my able associate for a number of years has been breaking fasts on whole foods for several years and finds that in most cases it is far superior to breaking the fast on juices, as was formerly advised. She reasoned that animals in the wild have no juicers or blenders and therefore have to break their fasts naturally on whole foods. Why should man be an exception?

Using her knowledge of physiology, she further reasoned that the bulk in the food is necessary to promote both peristalsis and mixing contractions in the stomach and intestines. Bulk is also necessary to promote secretion of the digestive juices of the stomach and intestines. The bulk of the food touching the stomach and intestinal walls is the *stimulus* for muscular contractions as well as for proper digestive secretions. Because of this, solid food is digested and handled more efficiently than juices. It is held in the stomach and intestines long enough for proper digestion and absorption, whereas juices, lacking this bulk are hurried along the digestive tract. Lacking in bulk, juices do not occasion strong peristaltic waves and do not elicit the gastrocolic reflex as strongly as solid foods. Because of these facts when the fast is broken on juices the first bowel movement after a fast is delayed. When solid foods are used to break the fast, bowel movements are reestablished much earlier.

Chewing of food is necessary both psychologically and physiologically. Another advantage of breaking the fast with solids is that the faster does not become bloated and over-filled with fluids. Taking the bulk with the food prevents overeating and the post faster is more satisfied with his meals. When fruit or vegetable juices are used there is a loss of vitamins and nutriments by oxidation no matter how carefully nor how quickly the juice is prepared. Some fasters are afraid to drink the juice rapidly and take one sip every fifteen minutes. By the time they have taken four ounces of juice in this manner almost two hours have passed with the juice oxidizing all the while. Breaking the fast with four ounces of whole orange, a section at a time may be eaten with a minimum of oxidation.

The fast may be broken at any time of the day or night that hunger recurs. If broken in advance of the return of hunger, it may be broken arbitrarily at 8:00 a.m. A number of techniques for breaking the fast have been worked out. Indeed, almost every man who conducts fasts has his own favorite plan. The main need is wholesome food; but not too much of it.

Dr. Crane, previously mentioned in these pages, used to give a faster an orange to eat in breaking the fast. The well-known Henry Lindlahr, M.D., now deceased, formerly of Chicago and Elmhurst, Illinois, who was director of the College of Natural Therapeutics in Chicago, broke fasts with a handful of pop corn. His reason for this was that the corn served as a broom to sweep out the digestive tract. In any case the pop corn did no harm.

The care exercised in breaking a fast is commonly proportioned to the length of a fast. Let me describe the plan we now employ. Assume that the fast has extended beyond fourteen days. We start the faster with four ounces of whole orange (weighed without the peeling) every two hours during the first day feeding is resumed. We prefer to start feedings at eight o'clock in the morning and stop at six in the evening—obviously this can be done only when the fast is broken in advance of the return of hunger. When hunger returns the fast should be broken without regard to the time. No harm is done, however, if the faster waits until 8:00 a.m. should hunger recur at midnight or in the wee hours of the morning.

On the second day, we give the faster eight ounces of orange or any other fresh juice fruit in season (weighed without rind or peeling) every two hours. A different fruit may be used for each feeding. If a faster has no desire for a feeding he is advised to skip a feeding or two. But this rarely occurs as it does when the fast is broken on juices. There is no compulsory amount of food he must take during this period.

On the third day we give twelve ounces of whole orange or melon for breakfast, two or three oranges, or two or three tomatoes, depending on their size for lunch, and three or four oranges for the evening meal. After the third day it is no longer necessary to weigh the food as the body again becomes accustomed to handling food. Instead of oranges, the third day, an equivalent amount of grapefruit or other juicy fruit in season may be given. The particular food given is not so important as avoiding overfeeding the faster. These fruits should be fresh, well ripened, and well chewed. Any tendency of the feeder to hurried eating should be discouraged.

On the fourth day the faster gets a small breakfast composed of citrus fruits or one or two other fresh fruits, or melon in season; at noon, a vegetable salad without salt, oil, vinegar, lemon juice or dressing of any kind, and one cooked nonstarchy vegetable. For the evening meal I feed fruit again. This meal should be light, but may be slightly larger than the breakfast.

On the fifth day, another fruit breakfast; a salad, two cooked green vegetables and a baked potato or a protein (small quantity) at noon, and a fruit meal again in the evening. I permit a glass of sour milk, (made from unpasteurized milk) at this fruit meal for those who are not vegetarians.

On the sixth day the feeding is about the same as on the fifth day, except that the amounts are increased. By the end of the first week the faster should be able to take normal amounts of food. No between meal eating is permitted and no eating in the evening before retiring is allowed. Three meals a day, simple and composed of fresh foods, constitute the best plan of feeding following a fast. If, later, the individual desires to adopt a two-meal or a one-meal plan of eating, this is best done after he has acquired some weight.

Bed rest should be continued through the first week of eating and activity begun very gradually. It is common for the faster to want to become active as soon as he resumes eating. This is unwise. He is not so strong and he does not have the endurance he thinks he has. Also activity retards his gain in weight if he has fasted to add weight.

Some fasters want to take long walks as soon as eating is resumed. Such activity is often over indulged to the extend that it often retards recuperation and causes the individual's weight to stand still. One must take it easy for a few days before resuming normal activities.

If the fast has been less than two weeks in duration, breaking it may be done with eight ounces of whole fruit every two hours the first day, then the preceding program followed from there. Less caution is required in breaking a short fast of this kind, and activity may be resumed sooner after a short fast.

All of this is true, of course, in those individuals who are in a fair state of health. If there is need for added rest and for light eating for some time after breaking a short fast, the faster must be guided by the judgment of his adviser.

But the most important advice, for all fasters at the breakfast point, is this: *Go slowly!*

13

Can Fasting Keep You Well?

There is no such miracle as permanent recovery in the sense that we can become so healthy we need give no further attention to our health. Nor is there any such thing as permanent weight reduction in the sense that we can eat all we want and stay thin.

Caring for the needs of life to secure health and proper weight maintenance is a constant *Hygienic* responsibility. We have all the health we deserve and no more.

No genuine recovery can be made until the cause of the impairment of health is removed and no perpetuation of the recovery is possible except upon a basis of continued avoidance of the causes of ill health.

To remain well requires that we live in a way to perpetuate good health. Whatever breaks down health in the first place will do so again, if it is returned to after health has been restored. Fasting will not provide man with a license to debauch himself. Fasting followed by gourmandizing is stupid. The drunk who sobers up can and will get drunk again if he returns to drink. If he ignores the drink he will not again become drunk.

When a man learns his limitations in food consumption, and respects these, he will remain well. If he habitually oversteps these, he will build disease and no plan of *immunization* can prevent him from becoming ill.

A return to coffee and tobacco, to alcohol and poisoned soft-drinks, to overwork and late hours, to unventilated bedrooms and slothfulness, to overeating and the conventional diet, in a word, to the old disease-producing way of life will build again physical troubles that have subsided with fasting. The only basis upon which to establish and maintain high-level health is supplied by first-class living habits.

What are the causes of disease? Any and all habits of mind and body that use up nerve energy in excess. Whatever factor or combination of factors that produces enervation is a cause of disease. If we squander our energies in many ways, we will enervate ourselves and begin the evolution of more disease. It is inevitable, under such circumstances, that elimination shall be checked and waste accumulate in the body.

Thus it becomes apparent that a corrected pattern of life involves far more than a mere change in eating habits. The sexual life, emotional life, working life, domestic life and all other elements of living that make up the complex of our lives are each vital to health. Each habit must be ordered and controlled in keeping with the unchanging laws that govern the living organism.

Fasting results in a radical cleansing of the fluids and tissues of the body, but it cannot prevent the subsequent fouling of these same fluids and tissues brought on by the return to overeating patterns. We can stay well only so long as we live in a manner to maintain and increase the gains we have made.

If we cannot return to these old and discarded routines, what should we eat? Can we continue at least in buying the ordinary dishes of average families?

To answer that I must point out certain facts of modern food that affect all of our civilization. We are living in an over-processed age, in terms of our diet. Everything is refined, stripped of its essential food values, baked, fried, cooked, over-stuffed. This is one of the great perils of our age. It is also one of the great problems of any person who wants to live on natural foods.

Natural products, coming from the hands of nature before they have been tampered with by the processors and refiners, are the one source that has consistently proved, throughout the ages, dependable both for man and animal. In spite of claims that processed and packaged substitutes for foods are as good or better than nature's products, the fact remains that no truly adequate substitutes for the products of nature have been discovered and prepared in the laboratories. The acid test of a food, it seems to me, is its fitness to serve the nutritive needs of the human organism just coming off a prolonged fast.

In all of my experience with feeding I have found nothing turned out synthetically by foods manufacturers to equal the untouched products of garden, orchard and field. Processing removes vitally important minerals from the foods, and either removes or makes valueless some or all of the precious vitamins. Enzymes are destroyed and many of the amino acids of the proteins in the food are destroyed. (Amino acids are destroyed by heat.)

Because of the destruction of food values by cooking and the removal of essential food factors by processing and refining. I emphasize the importance of eating fresh, uncooked fruits and vegetables daily. Indeed, these foods should constitute no less than sixty percent of the daily diet. There can be no doubt that less protein will be required to supply the daily amino acid needs of the body if these are taken in the uncooked state.

Cooking also has the added disadvantage of leeching out much of the values of the food. Nourishment is lost in the juices that ooze from the foods in cooking; it is lost in the water in which the foods are boiled or steamed. Food values are evaporated by the high temperature and are chemically altered and rendered unusable as foods.

One should make it a rule, from which there should be no variations, to have one meal of fresh, uncooked fruit each day and at least one large raw vegetable salad daily. The salads commonly eaten are too small to meet our needs and are often made up of such things as mashed potatoes, boiled eggs, pickled olives and other such substances, to which is added a greasy dressing—but with little in the way of either fresh fruits or vegetables. Some of them contain a leaf or two of semi-wilted lettuce, a slice of half-ripened tomato, and dressing. Hardly enough to nourish a canary.

Salads of raw vegetables and meals of fresh fruits are essential sources of minerals and vitamins. These foods are more abundant in these food factors, and are as necessary to the nutrition of man as an abundance of green grass is essential to the horse or cow. He who partakes of these foods each day will have no need to add mineral concentrates and vitamin pills to his diet. These raw properties are the normal or natural sources of such food factors and nothing has yet been produced by the food chemists that can take their places.

Minerals are as essential to the formation and preservation of the body as proteins. They are important to the formation and maintenance of the blood, bones, teeth, muscles, glands, nerves. There is a continuous demand for these substances by the active organism. Each day some of the minerals are used and excreted and each day they must be replenished. But we are not able to supply the body with minerals by eating lime and scrap iron.

We are able to make use of minerals only in certain forms as these are prepared for our use by the processes of plant life. The drug store cannot supply us with any just-as-good minerals to replace those that are removed from our foods in the refining processes. Nor do we get our best supply of minerals from powdered egg shells and bone meal. From the vegetable kingdom comes our best mineral supply.

Proteins are abundant in nature and there is rarely an excuse for protein deficiency in this country. Every food that grows contains proteins so that in eating natural foods one receives these from several sources each day. Whatever essential amino acids may be lacking in one protein is sure to be compensated by other amino acids in the other proteins of the diet.

Nuts are one of the finest sources of the best and most adequate proteins. Green leaves contain small quantities of most excellent proteins. There are proteins in bananas, dates, figs, legumes, cereals and in a hundred other foods eaten daily.

After a fast, when the body's food reserve has been somewhat depleted, the three food essentials that are most needed are proteins, minerals and vitamins. These are best secured from the sources indicated.

Canned foods, preserved foods, processed and refined foods, adulterated foods, sulphured fruits, white flour, white sugar, white rice, constitute **poor** materials with which to build healthy tissue.

Man's need for fats or oils is not as great as may be supposed, but he does require a small daily amount of these and he instinctively seeks such foods. In many seeds, such as sunflower seed, peanuts, soy beans, nuts and in the avocado, olive, and other fruits, nature has packaged an abundant supply of the finest and tastiest oils. We do not need to seek for refined oils in order to supply the fat needs of our body. Indeed, the oils stored in natural foods are associated with minerals and vitamins, so that they are far superior to the refined fats and oils on the market.

What I have written here of fats and oils applies with equal force to sugars and starches. In their natural state, these food factors are ideally associated with minerals and vitamins and they are best eaten in the unrefined state. Syrups and refined sugars are devoid of minerals and vitamins and are poor foods. The sweet fruits: dates, figs, raisins, sweet grapes, well-ripened bananas, persimmons, and similar products are the finest and best sources of sugars and should be eaten as fruits rather than as fragmented food particles produced by manufacturers of refined products— out of a tin can.

In summarizing, any return to the overeating that may have characterized the pre-fasting way of life will quickly build a state of ill health. Learn to be moderate in eating habits. One of the best aids to moderation is the eating of whole natural foods. We are practically forced to overeat when we try to live on a diet that is composed predominantly of processed and refined foods. We do this in an effort to secure the food needs that are lacking in these foodless foods.

Fasting cannot keep you well. Only sound habits will do so.

14

Rejuvenation through Fasting

She was sixty years of age and had suffered for years with a minor heart ailment. I put her on a fast of three weeks. She rested in bed while the fast was in progress. At the end of her fast she remarked: "My heart feels so rested! It is so quiet I hardly know I have one in my body."

This represented an improvement in the condition of the woman that was genuine and lasting. Overweight when she started, with high blood pressure, she lost twenty pounds and her blood pressure was greatly reduced, lifting a great burden from her heart.

Her general feeling of vigor and well-being matched the improvement of her heart. Her former sleeplessness had given way to restful nightly repose. The improvement in her bowel action was as marked as that of her heart function. Certainly her improved youthfulness of appearance and the brightness of her eyes, spoke volumes for the rejuvenating effects of her physiological rest.

Anyone experienced with fasting has seen great numbers of such instances of physical rejuvenation achieved by means of the fast. The mental improvements commonly match the physical improvements. Occasional restoration of hearing in ears that have been deaf for years, improved vision, discarding glasses that have been worn for years (but rarely restoration of sight to blind eyes), increased acuteness of the senses of taste and smell, restoration of ability to sense delicate flavors, recovery of the sense of feeling in instances of sensory paralysis, stepped-up vigor, increased mental powers, loss of weight, greatly increased functional vigor, with better digestion and better bowel action, clear sparkling eyes, clearing of the complexion with a restoration of youthful bloom, the disappearance of some of the finer lines of the face, reduced blood pressure, better heart action, reduction of enlarged prostate, sexual rejuvenation—these and many other evidences of rejuvenation are seen by everyone who has a wide experience with fasting.

Fasting can bring about a virtual rebirth, a revitalization of the organism. As the fast progresses, all of the cells of the body undergo refinement and there is a removal from the protoplasm of the cells of stored foreign substances (metaplasmic materials) so that the cells become more youthful and function more efficiently.

Some of these stored materials are highly toxic and have long remained in the fatty cells and in the cells of the connective tissues which have been appropriately termed the "dumping ground of the body" to get them out of the circulation. Freeing the tissues of such materials renders the body more efficient as a physiologic mechanism. Besides the renovation that fasting enables the body to undergo, there is created a potential for better function which continues long after the fast has been broken.

Wear and waste with repair and replenishment are continuous and almost simultaneous processes in all living structures. The one is a building up, the other a tearing down. The two processes have received the technical name of *metabolism* as described above, and are called respectively, *anabolism*, the building up, and *catabolism* which is the tearing down. Catabolism predominates during periods of activity; anabolism during periods of rest and repose.

Anabolism may be defined as the process by which the body is repaired, reinvigorated and prepared for renewed activity. It is the dominant process during periods of active growth; it is somewhat slowed down in age.

Fasting has been shown to result in an accelerated metabolism, with the emphasis after the fast is broken, on the anabolic, or constructive phase. This is to say: the general cleansing of the body renews the building-up process of life. It is true that under experimental conditions, this improvement of the process of life is not lasting. But this has been due, in great measure, to the failure of experimenters to follow up the fasts with anything other than a speedy return to conventional modes of living.

A man's age is the duration of his life. When we use the term age to mean several aspects of that life, the stage of one's development (physiological age), the mental development attained (psychological age) or any other such term or phrase which signifies something other than chronological age, we are confusing age with body condition or with stages of growth and development.

When we say that a man is old at forty and that another man is young at seventy we actually refer to the physical and mental states of the two men and not to their ages. The suggestion that we use the phrase "functional age" in speaking of an individual and make no reference to his birthdays is based on the same confusion.

It is true that birthdays do not tell the condition of one's body, nor do they tell how well developed the mind may be, but conditions are related to age only incidentally and are not essential parts of age. A man of seventy may be youthful in physical condition or in mental outlook, or a man of forty may be old in condition, flaccid and depressed, but the first is still seventy years old and the other is only forty years of age.

Knowing these things, we may ignore the objection often offered that we are "trying to set the clock back." The changes called "aging" that take place in the body are not related so much to the clock of time as to causes totally unrelated to time as such.

If the clock had casual relation to "aging," we should expect the man of seventy to show all the signs of "aging" that are common to this time of life, and the man of forty to present all the signs of "youthfulness" that are common then. That we so frequently see these facts in reverse should cause us to question the assumption that the condition of the body is irrevocably related to the number of years we have lived. We should not find it difficult to understand that we "age" in time, but time is not the cause of the "aging" process. Think of the stone worn away by water. It changes in time, but time does not wear it away. The water wears it away. The process of wearing away the stone takes time—time is not the wearing process.

Two stones subjected to the same amount of water-wearing, will wear away at different rates, depending on their respective hardness and density. For this same reason, two men, under the same amount of impairing influences will "age at different rates," depending on the resistance each offers to the causes of impairment.

A stone will wear faster or slower depending on the amount of water that flows over it; wearing slowly if only a small amount of water washes its surface, wearing faster if much water flows over it. In the same way, a man will "age" slowly or rapidly, depending on the amount of impairing influence to which he is subjected.

Carrying our comparison a bit further: if we can conceive of a self-repairing rock being worn away and then having the water cease flowing over it, we'd see the rock repair itself and restore much of its former substance, and would witness a process similar to that which takes place in the human organism (which is self-repairing) when the causes of "aging" are removed.

The body is capable of tearing down some of its damaged structures and replacing these with new structures; it is capable of renewing its cells, of casting off its accumulated burdens and of repairing much of its damages. Unlike the lifeless rock, the living organism is capable of taking an active hand in its affairs and doing something constructive.

Man is constituted for longer and better life than he now enjoys. He should live considerably many more years than he now does. And he should enjoy the possession of full health and vigor. He should not fall apart at sixty or earlier. The fact is that, barring death by accident or killing, as in war, human beings die of disease. If we live in such a manner as to prevent the evolution of disease, we not only may live much longer than is now thought possible, but we may live in full possession of all our mental and physical powers.

Aging has been defined as "the accumulation of body changes that increase one's chances of dying with the passage of time." This simply means that aging is the slow accumulation of pathological (diseased) changes in the organs and tissues of the body. It signifies the accumulation of damages to the structures of the body and a slow impairment of the functions of life. Old age is simply one more chronic disease. This is the reason we may *age* early or late, and why some men are younger at seventy than others are at forty.

Age takes place in time but is not caused by time. It is not important, therefore, that means be found of determining accurately one's physiological age. What is important is that we find and recognize the causes of the aging process. Remove the cause of aging; and the physiological age takes care of itself.

It is claimed that no one knows precisely what the body changes that constitute aging consist of, or what exactly the changes might be. The experiments of the noted French scientist, Dr. Alexis Carrell, author of *Man, the Unknown*, in keeping fragments of a chicken heart alive for many years, revealed that they aged when not kept free of their own cell waste. In other words, they aged as a consequence of the accumulation, in the culture medium in which they were kept, of their own metabolic waste.

If these wastes were regularly washed away, so that the cells were not poisoned by them, the chicken heart did not age. We have indications again that aging is the result of chronic toxic saturation. This important finding has received all too little attention, perhaps because there was no way to exploit it.

Carrell's experiments and many more like them have led to the conclusion by some authorities that the cells are potentially *immortal*. Normally they continue to divide and redivide, but they do not die. From this viewpoint death would seem to be abnormal. What we observe, however, under all ordinary conditions of life, is that the cells do age and they do die in great numbers. To go on living indefinitely, all conditions must be favorable.

If the cells are potentially ageless, as is now believed by scientists, and the complex body ages, then it is evident that one of two things is true. Either the functional specialization of cell groups—the organs of the body— is inadequate, or there is some lack of coordination of the cell groups in the body. Perhaps there may be both. If one or both of the propositions is true, the question becomes: is the inadequacy of specialization or the inadequacy of coordination a primary state of life or is it a result of ascertainable and removable causes? If it is primary, we cannot hope to prevent, for more than a brief span, the aging process, which seems to set in, in most cases, rather early in life. If it is due to avoidable and removable causes, as seems likely, we should be able to do much to prevent aging.

At least in many of the lower forms of life numerous experiments have demonstrated that not only can the aging process be indefinitely held off, but also that it can be reversed and youthfulness restored.

For more than fifteen years, Professor C. M. Child of the University of Chicago did research on aging in animals. His results revealed that periodic fasting is generally conducive to rejuvenescence.

In certain species of insects he found that, with abundant food, insects pass through their whole life-history in three to four weeks, but when the food is greatly reduced or the insects are forced to fast, they may continue active and young for at least three years. His conclusion was that "partial starvation (fasting) inhibits senescence. The starveling is brought back from an advanced age to the beginning of postembryonic life; it is almost reborn."

Child pointed out that in the organic world generally, rejuvenescence is but the regular or ordinary process of cell renewal that is in continuous operation throughout the life of every organism.

The failure to maintain youthfulness is due to causes that prevent the ideal operation of the regular renewal process. Any removal of these hindering causes, at any age, results in a movement in the direction of renewed youthfulness.

Professor Child's experiments led Anton J. Carlson, Professor of Physiology in the same university, to experiment for years with both fasting and feeding, in an effort to determine how much rejuvenation could be brought about in man by the same means that result in rejuvenation of lower forms of life. He was convinced that he found evidence of the rejuvenating effects of fasting in man. Unfortunately his experiments with human subjects were all too few and most of them were performed on more or less youthful subjects.

Frederick Hoelzel, who did much of the fasting that Professor Carlson observed, thinks that the possibilities of rejuvenescence progressively decrease as age advances and that little rejuvenation may be expected after the age of thirty-five. On this I am compelled to take issue with him. I think that his observations in this field have been too narrowly limited to justify setting any such arbitrary limit to the possibilities of human rejuvenation. Thirty-five is not a fixed landmark in human life. It is not an age in which irreversible changes have been made in human tissues.

It must be recognized that there exist sharply defined limits to the possibilities of human rejuvenation. There are irreversible changes in the tissues of man's body and trying to undo them is like attempting to grow a new leg after one has been lost. In many of the lower forms of animal life, some of them very complex animals, the ability to grow new members or internal organs (even new heads, brains and eyes) is possible, and the possibilities of rejuvenation are much greater in such organisms than in the higher forms. But a greater degree of rejuvenation is possible in man than we have heretofore thought.

We may accept as true the claim that the greater the amount and extent of pathological changes that have taken place in the body of man, the less are his possibilities of rejuvenation. We may agree with Hoelzel that the older one grows, the less are his possibilities of renewing youthfulness. Yet some of the most remarkable examples of rejuvenation I have witnessed have been in men and women past sixty. Without the least desire to discount the value of the work done by laboratory experimenters with fasting, I think that I am justified in saying that these observations have been too narrowly restricted to enable the laboratory workers to give us the final word.

Yet I do not think the greatest possibilities of the fast are in the rejuvenation of old men and women. Its possibility for reversing the process of senescence in younger men and women so that the aging process is slowed down, represents an equally important role. If we can employ fasting to prevent damaging changes in vital organs, by periodically freeing the body of its toxic load, and by giving the organs of life much needed rest, we should be able to accomplish far more lasting good in preventing aging than in seeking rejuvenation of the aged.

Some investigators stress the evanescent character of the rejuvenating effects of fasting and have taken the position that they are not worth the effort required to bring them about. To this objection there are two important replies.

First: A temporary regeneration is all that is needed to remove many structural defects and to improve the functioning efficiency of the organism. The removal of the toxic load is not evanescent and this is vitally important to the future of the organism.

Second: In making their investigations, as already noted, these research men have guaranteed the evanescent character of the gains made by the readiness with which they have returned the subjects of the experiments to their prior toxogenic ways of life.

In 1960, Tara Singh of India underwent a 48-day fast for political reasons. He was seventy-six years of age and his physicians gave it as their belief, after examining him, that his period of abstinence had "increased his life span by at least ten years."

This statement of his physicians, issued from New Delhi, added that the fasting period had "relieved illness from which he was suffering." While the improvement of the health of Singh was a by-product of his fast, it is both interesting and significant to find that his physicians are candid enough to give credit to the period of abstinence for the benefits to his health. It is usual for physicians to discredit all reports of benefits resulting from fasting. Perhaps this incident represents a turning point in their attitude.

We hope that physicians will soon come to recognize in fasting a natural means of rejuvenation that is actually superior to gland grafts, the mascerated organs of unborn lambs, and the use, generally, of animal and insect products, which, so far, have provided no genuine rejuvenation. Perhaps this change in attitude can lead to a recognition of the fact that whatever rejuvenation an organism is capable of effecting, is the product of the operation of intrinsic forces and processes under favorable conditions, and not a forced state resulting from exotic impositions. Recovery of health (this is to say, clearing up of pathological states) and rejuvenation may yet be seen to be one and the same process.

Brown-Sequard's seminal fluid rejuvenator; Steinach's subcutaneous division of the *vas deferens* (the duct or tube carrying the secretion of the testes), supposed to result in rejuvenation; Voronoff's monkey gland transplantation; Brinkley's goat gland transplantation; Funk's vitamin rejuvenation plan all having failed, perhaps we can turn our attention to a more rational approach to the problems created by aging.

If we can see in fasting a means of enabling the body to free itself, not alone of its accumulated toxic load, but also of its burden of accumulated abnormal changes in its tissues, we can use this means of rejuvenation to great advantage.

Recognizing its limitations and not expecting the impossible, we may still find in the fast an avenue perhaps not to eternal youth but to a protracted youth that endures long into what we once considered—old age!

15

Fasting to Gain Weight

Almost everybody can understand fasting to lose weight, but it may be difficult for many of the readers to understand fasting to gain weight. However, it is a common experience with fasting, that in a great number of cases, the first weight gains made, follow a fast.

Overfeeding with loss of weight is a familiar pattern; every day we meet underweight people who are eating valiantly to gain weight and they complain that the more they eat the more they lose. They try first one weight-gaining diet and then another but remain thin or grow thinner. The overfed organism is often undernourished to a degree that reveals itself in rapid emaciation.

Food and nutrition are not synonymous. One is not nourished in proportion to the amount of food ingested, but in proportion to how much one digests and assimilates. When digestion and assimilation are impaired, overeating in an effort to put on weight defeats its purpose. Emaciation is due to impairment of health, rarely to lack of food. The emaciation is commonly proportionate to the extent of the impairment of health. What such patients need is not more food but a properly functioning de-toxified system able to digest and assimilate food. Given this they have no difficulty in gaining weight.

Because fasting results in a rejuvenation of assimilation, it commonly enables chronically underweight patients to gain weight where everything else fails. Naturally they lose weight during the fast, but they regain more after the fast is broken than they lose during the fast. This is in harmony with both experience and experiment in the animal kingdom.

Experimental fasts have demonstrated that after a fast less food is required to maintain physical energies, physiological activities, nitrogen balance, and weight, because fasting produces a more efficient physiological machine. This is the reason that the emaciated person, who remains thin on the various "weight gaining" diets, commonly finds that after a fast he will gain weight on much less food than he has been in the habit of taking.

From long observation farmers report the following. If a pig smaller than other members of the litter because of insufficient milk is taken from the litter and fed adequately, it grows more rapidly than the others in the litter, catching up with and even passing them in size.

Osborn, Mendel and Thomson, three standard authorities in dietetics and biochemistry, in a series of classical experiments, confirmed these observations under test conditions. They found that the growth which is resumed after an arrest by insufficient food, proceeds at a more rapid pace than usual, attaining, for a time, a magnitude which they ascribe to an excess of compensation.

A similar phenomenon is observed to occur after a fast by the emaciated. The period of physiological rest provided by the fast, results in better digestion, better assimilation and a better and more economical use of food. It has been shown that fasting results in an intense nitrogen hunger and, at the same time, a greatly increased capacity to utilize nitrogen. This provides for the production of a better type of tissue than the fatty tissues which result from overeating on starches, sugars and fats.

Reduced to simplest terms, this means that the body calls for and utilizes proteins more readily and thus puts on a very different type of flesh from that which results from stuffing on sugars, starches and fats. Where this latter type of eating often results in a gain of weight it is nothing more significant than the laying on of pounds of useless fat. Protein-built tissue, on the other hand, is good, sound and useful tissue and provides for a much better appearance of body. It is important in gaining weight to gain it properly and healthfully.

There is a wealth of evidence to show that metabolism is accelerated by fasting, a fact which can only mean a more efficient turn-over of nutritive materials. Metabolism is the term applied to the overall process by which foods are transformed into flesh and by which the used up substances are disassimilated. It is especially the building up phase of metabolism (called anabolism) that is accelerated by the fast. The fact is undeniable that after a fast the tissues are more receptive to food elements and readily assimilate and utilize vitamins, minerals and proteins, even in individuals who failed to do so before.

In well-fed, indeed over-fed America, we meet few emaciated individuals who are underweight from eating too little food. Their lack of weight is most often due to failure to digest and assimilate the food they eat. Such individuals need not more food, but added capacity to digest and assimilate their food. Added capacity can be acquired only by remedying the functional and organic impairments that are responsible for the crippled states of their nutrition.

It is rarely possible to do this so long as the patient continues to eat his regular daily ration of what he considers "good nourishing food." The curious fact is that many of these patients will gain weight if they eat much less than they are in the habit of taking. They are especially helped by a fast of proper duration.

Subjects with poor nutrition commonly have a poor appetite. It is usual to assume that their nutrition is poor because they do not eat enough; whereas, the opposite is true; reduced eating is the result of poor nutrition. When the food is not used, the body cuts off demand—hunger ceases. Nature is wiser than we are in these matters. Not more food, but more capacity to use food, is what is needed.

Fasting sharpens appetite. Not only do these patients have keener relish for food and a stronger demand for food, following a fast, but they have better digestion and increased capacity to assimilate their food. They also gain weight, and in many instances they gain it rapidly. I have seen amazing gains of this kind and have seen individuals long underweight gain so much that they had to reverse the field and begin to reduce.

Exceptions to this experience are seen almost wholly, in those long, skinny individuals who suffer with what is commonly referred to as nervous exhaustion or nervous collapse. Such people are benefited by the fast but they rarely gain rapidly after the fast. The profound depression of the nervous system in these patients, and the consequent depression of their functions, require an extended period of careful control not alone of their eating, but of their total way of life, to restore functioning power to the point where they are able to put on solid weight.

How long should the underweight individual fast to secure improvement in his nutritional processes? There is no absolute undeviating answer. Each case is different as the condition of each patient is different. In some cases a fast of ten days to two weeks will prove adequate. In others much longer fasts may be called for. A short fast is rarely enough to secure the correction of the defects of the nutritional processes needed to enable the chronically underweight person to gain weight. Here, as elsewhere, the fast should be taken under competent supervision and the judgment of the supervisor respected.

Since most cases of underweight with which we deal in this country are due, not to insufficient food, but to incapacity to digest and assimilate food, it is essential that all causes of impaired nutrition be discovered and removed. Fasting should not be expected to result in a great improvement of the body's ability to digest and assimilate the food eaten, if the patient continues with practices that perpetuate the impairment. Rest, in order that nerve energy may be recuperated, is also vital.

Following the fast, it is not wise to overeat on foods that are commonly thought to constitute a weight gaining diet. On the contrary, the requirements of good nutrition are best met with a diet consisting of at least sixty percent fresh leafy vegetables and fresh fruits. Canned vegetables and fruits are not to be considered as food with which to follow up a fast. The protein and carbohydrate content of the diet may make up the other forty percent, with emphasis on the better class proteins.

In addition to a greatly improved diet, every other healthful factor that enables us to build and maintain high level health should be made an integral part of the daily life of the individual. Daily exercise, an abundance of fresh air, sunbaths where these are at all possible, an abundance of rest and sleep, emotional poise and freedom from all devitalizing habits will greatly assist in building weight and in producing the kind of tissue that is desirable.

It will be noted that this advice is similar to that given to the overweight individual who has fasted and is desirous of building wholesome flesh. The fact is that a normal life builds a normal condition. Normal weight has its basis in good health and in first class habits of life. The genuine needs of both types of patients are the same.

16

Should Children Fast?

I am often asked about fasting for infants and young children. Is it safe? Should it be attempted? The answer is that children often know instinctively when to fast—and for how long.

Let me cite the case of an anxious mother who consulted me about her young son who appeared to be, so far as he was able to carry it out, on a permanent fast.

"My child simply won't eat," the mother told me. "I have to force him. I make him come to the dining table. I make him eat. Unless I force him, he won't touch his food."

"Why not leave him alone until he gets hungry?" I suggested.

"He never gets hungry. He would starve to death."

Many mothers face this problem with their children. Few subjects are more talked about—with more misinformation—than the feeding of children. We hear about loss of appetite, undernourishment, and underweight in children, and the fact that a child may be suffering from eating too much is rarely guessed. Yet in forty years I have never seen a child "starve to death" because it refused to eat. I have watched hundreds of them go without food until they become hungry, and I have never seen one that was not soon raising old Ned for food.

In the case above, I persuaded the mother to give her boy a chance to get hungry to see if he would not do the same.

"Wait," I told her. "When he is hungry he will tell you."

He did. When the food vanished, when he was not forced to swallow more than his body demanded or required, he soon began to want to eat normally.

In a few days we had a happy mother and a less unruly boy. She reported: "Dick is now the first one to the table and we no longer have to force him to swallow every mouthful."

Leave the child alone when he refuses food. It is certain that he will become hungry within a reasonable time and will demand food. Abstinence from food is the surest and best *appetizer* available. It is better than coercion, which tends to create resistance. It is better than tempting them with dainty dishes and flavored and sweetened dishes to appeal to jaded appetites. It is better than feeding vitamins or giving tonics.

Let the child go without food until a natural demand for food is made in the form of hunger and it will be content with plain fare. There will be no need to tempt it with special dishes. No chocolate will have to be added to its milk, ice cream will not have to be substituted for wholesome food, tidbits and palate ticklers will no longer be found necessary. Why should a child, any more than an adult, be forced to eat? If there is no physiological demand for food, why should it be forced upon the child?

With the majority of well-meaning adults, when they undertake to coax a child to eat, the food with which they tempt the child is usually unsuitable. It is commonly the worst possible selection that is responsible for the loss of desire for food. It is ruinous to the character of the child to bribe it by offering money, a toy, a trip to the movies, or to hold out other inducements to it to eat when there is no natural demand for food. Such means of inducing a child to eat lead inevitably to overeating.

Overeating results in temporary loss of desire for food. Candy or cookies between meals destroys the desire to eat. Mothers who permit children to eat between meals should not be surprised if they are not hungry when meal time arrives. Children often develop "poor appetites" because of the unsuitable character of their diet. McCarrison who made original study in the field of dietetics—and later reported on the Hunzas—says: "It seems to me that 'loss of appetite' is one of the most fundamental signs of vitamin deprivation. It is a protective sign: the first signal of impending disaster."

After a brief period of abstinence it should be understood that when the amount of food taken is reduced, the vitamin needs of the body are correspondingly reduced—the diet of the child should be changed. Give them more fruits and vegetables (fresh and uncooked) and less cereal, bread, potatoes, cookies, pies and candies. Eliminate all soft drinks. Mothers will no longer have to worry about vitamins for their children if they supply them with the natural sources of vitamins.

I quote McCarrison again: "There are no more important ingredients of a properly constituted diet than fruits and vegetables, for they contain vitamins of every class, recognized and unrecognized."

Why feed your child a baked apple, when the uncooked apple is more nutritious and far more tasty? Why give it candy made of white sugar, synthetic colors and flavors, wood glue, and other unwholesome substances, as long as there are dates, figs, bananas and other sweet fruits, which are more tasty and more wholesome? There is more vitamin value in a stalk of celery or a head of bibb lettuce than in all the vitamin pills in the drug store. An orange or a peach will provide wholesome nutriment for your child. A dish of ice cream is about as unwholesome as anything he can take. Soft drinks are poisonous and unfit to swallow. More care in feeding the child will give it better health and save parents much anxiety and expense. *Children's diseases are parents' mistakes.*

Children lack desire for food when they are ill. Enervated children, with gastritis, enlarged tonsils and adenoids, constipation, diarrhea, feverishness, will express no demand for food. They should be permitted to skip a meal or several meals, as circumstances warrant, and no effort should be made to force them or coax them to eat.

Any unusual excitement of children, even a trip or a picnic, may use up so much nerve energy that indigestion is produced. Symptoms of indigestion may range all the way from irritability, restlessness, tossing during sleep, bad breath, "growing pains," white lines around the mouth, to fever, gastric pains, nausea, vomiting and great discomfort evidenced by extreme restlessness. When such symptoms are present no food should be given. If children with indigestion are fed and treated in the customary manner, the state of the stomach and intestinal tract is likely to become putrescent, laying the ground work for possible serious disease.

Infants become enervated from being handled too much, from being carried about, from having their rest broken, from being subjected to noise—too much commotion in the house—by being nursed and trundled too much, by being played with and excited too much, by being subjected to too much heat and cold, by being fed too much, by being drugged for symptoms and inoculated for *disease prevention.*

In dealing with the child, of course, competent *Hygienic* guidance should be sought and followed. When a baby is enervated, the digestive function falters; indigestion with fermentation and putrefaction of food results. The putrescence thus evolved irritates the lining membrane of the stomach and intestine. The membrane of the stomach, bowel or air passage becomes a site of supplementary or compensatory excretion, the eliminating process being named, according to its location, as a cold, bronchitis, gastritis, diarrhea, etc. There may be a slight feverish condition accompanied by a "sick stomach" or a slight cough. The baby is restless and uneasy, sleepless, fretful. The restlessness is likely to be interpreted as hunger and the child may be fed.

If the food is discontinued at once the slight indigestion quickly ends. The restlessness and fretfulness subside. If it is fed and handled—many parents walk the floor with sick infants—the irritableness, fretfulness and feverishness increase. If this program is continued, vomiting and diarrhea may ensue and the symptom-complex may be named enteritis, cholera infantum, colitis or dysentery. If the lungs are selected as fontanels through which to excrete the excess toxin, the symptom-complex may be named pneumonia. If eruptions appear on the skin, the disease will be named as hives, measles, scarlet fever, or smallpox.

"In childhood," wrote Dr. Oswald, "chronic dyspepsia is in nearly all cases the effect of chronic medication. Indigestion is not an hereditary complaint. A dietetic sin *per excessum*, a quantitative surfeit with sweet meats and pastry, may derange the digestive process for a few hours or so but the trouble passes by with the holidays. Lock up the short-cakes, administer a glass of cold water, and, my life for yours, that on Monday morning the little glutton will be ready to climb the steepest hill in the country. But stuff him with liver pills, drench him with cough syrup, and paregoric, and in a month or two he will not be able to satisfy the cravings of the inner boy without 'assisting nature' with a patent stimulant."

Babies and young children are prone to develop spasms as a consequence of severe indigestion. Each paroxysm scares the wits out of the parents, although it is usual for the youngster to be as well as ever the following day. As soon as the child recovers from the acute indigestion the spasms cease. The child with indigestion should not be fed.

Sometimes an older child, suffering with a mild feverish condition and inflammation of the digestive tract, will imagine that he is hungry and will demand food. This demand should not be acceded to. Feeding will only serve to increase its discomfort and retard his recovery. Hunger here is not genuine but most always only in the mind.

Gastritis is inflammation of the stomach. It may be immediately occasioned by over-feeding or eating freely of candy. When a baby becomes enervated from too much excitement, too much handling, overclothing, cold or in any other way, resulting in inhibition of excretion, a channel of compensatory or supplementary elimination is established through which to expel the accumulated toxin. The mucous membranes of the body are favorite channels through which fontannels—openings for use in discharge of excretions—are established for elimination purposes. If, as a consequence of local irritation, from overeating or candy eating, for example, the lining of the stomach is requisitioned to do vicarious duty, the baby has gastritis or indigestion. If the lining of the intestine or colon is chosen for supplementary services, a diarrhea will develop.

Perhaps a week or longer before the beginning of a fever, the observant mother may notice white specks in the bowel movements of her baby. These mean that the milk is not being well digested, perhaps due to overfeeding. The white specks may vary from small, white milk-curds throughout the stool to an amount of milk curd that makes up two-thirds to three-fourths of the stool. If the stool is gray and the consistency of putty, it is composed largely of undigested milk curd. If the stool is sour, this indicates fermentation. If the condition is corrected at this stage, nothing further will develop; but if not immediately corrected, inflammation of the stomach, small intestine and large intestine will develop.

If the indigestion is confined to the stomach, the child will be restless, irritable and feverish. At first there will be vomiting of food stuff. This is soon followed by vomiting of water and mucus, which may be slightly tinged with yellow. If food is withheld and water given in small doses, this crisis will end in a day to three or four days. The baby is likely to be thirsty and mothers are prone to mistake this for hunger, and to feed. The food will be vomited, even water is frequently ejected. Water, when given, should be warm and taken in small amounts. It is important for mothers to know that it is not a kindness on their part to feed a sick child. Food should always be withheld in stomach and intestinal diseases.

In short, while always acting under proper *Hygienic* direction with your child, do all that you can to let the natural tools of rest and peace and quiet restore the child if there is upset or illness—or even if it is only a question of how much he wants to eat.

For there are ways in which the instinctive wisdom of the infant or child in such matters may be far greater than we could possibly guess.

Fasting to Help You Get Well

In this section of the book we will examine more closely the uses of fasting for health. In general we will seek to give the reader a grasp of the nature of certain malfunctions and the way in which the fast can be of value. Again we stress the fact that fasting in itself has no force but rather it enables the body's organs and recuperative forces to turn their full energies upon the problem to be corrected.

This is the great secret power within.

17

Fasting in Acute Disease

"My baby is dying," a mother said over the telephone to a *Hygienist*.

It was the winter of 1927. The *Hygienist* was located in New York City, the mother called him from Nyack, N. Y.

"How do you know the baby is dying?"

The mother's reply was not heartening: "He has pneumonia. Five physicians have just held a consultation. It is their verdict my baby will die. There is nothing more that science can do."

"Let's fool them," said the *Hygienist*. "We could try to save her, you know—"

Over the phone the *Hygienist* then advised: "The first thing I want you to do is go to the table at the bedside of your baby and sweep all the boxes and bottles of drugs that are there into the waste basket. Next, open the window and let some fresh air into the room. Keep your baby warm, but give it some fresh air. Give the baby as much water as it wants, but no food and no more drugs."

Twenty years later this baby, grown to splendid young womanhood, was married and wedding pictures of her and her husband are prized possessions of the *Hygienist* who took over after the physicians had declared the baby would die.

It is not unusual to see patients recover after it has been declared that every thing had been done that science could do. This is so because the very things that science does are so often the causes of death. Drugs to suppress the cough and anodynes to stop the pain in the chest in pneumonia are frequent causes of death. Feeding in pneumonia is also dangerous. When in both pneumonia and pleurisy the patient is fed, not only is the toxemic supersaturation kept up, but the feeding prevents resolution, that is, it prevents the inflamed lung or pleura from returning to normal. This may result in abscess formation.

In the acute forms of disease—fevers and inflammations—the desire for food is absent, indicating that no food should be taken. There is an absence of the digestive juices, perhaps the walls of the digestive system are pouring out mucus profusely, as in acute gastritis or in typhoid fever, just as do the lining membranes of the nose and throat in a cold: the normal muscular movements of the digestive tract are suspended, and there is absence of power to digest food. Inflammation, pain and fever each suspend the digestive secretions and the movements of the stomach.

When the sufferer with acute disease is fed his pains and discomforts are increased, his temperature rises and his chances of recovery are reduced. In acute disease the digestive system is as little fit to digest food as the limbs are for locomotion. Both require rest. What good does it do for a man to take food, even the finest food, if he is unable to digest and assimilate it? Restless, suffering with nausea, not only with no desire for food, but actually loathing it, and not retaining it when swallowed, food certainly should not be taken. Forced feeding under such conditions is not nourishing, but depleting. Fasting is the only rational plan of care of a sick person presenting such symptoms.

A man is prostrated: everything tastes bitter to him, every little noise is agonizing and his mind wanders. His tongue is coated with a yellow-brown coat, the region over his stomach and bowels is sensitive, he vomits at short intervals, his temperature is above normal.

Should he be fed? Or could he be fed without adding to his discomfort and without danger?

Loss of desire for food is one of the first symptoms of acute disease. Go over the whole list—smallpox, typhoid fever, typhus fever, pneumonia, diphtheria, measles, cholera, and you realize that one of the first developments in these crises is the suspension of all desire for food. Wisely, nature cuts off all demand for food when it cannot be used. Fasting is a means of getting through such crises.

The fast is a temporary expedient by means of which the body achieves some of its urgently needed work, an expedient employed by the living organism to help it over many of the emergencies of life. It is almost correct to say that fasting and surgery are all that are of value in disease. But we can say this only if we recognize that the regular or ordinary elements of nature's great plan of *Hygiene* are as essential in illness as in health, except that their use must be modified to conform to the crippled powers of the organism.

Instead of fasting being a *cure*, it is an essential and integral part of the healing process. When the digestive system is prostrated and all desire for food is cut off, as it is in acute disease, we have an expedient that is as much a part of the remedial process, the process of restoration, as the concomitant prostration of the body as a whole that sends the sick person to bed. To be extremely precise, the fasting process is an actual part of the *remedial process* that we call disease.

Including surgery among the useful expedients in disease does not imply approval to all surgery performed today. Skillfully done, as much of it is, it is performed all too often for purely commercial motives rather than only when there is a legitimate reason for it. The fact will someday be known that fasting will obviate the supposed need for much of the surgery that is performed today. In stressing the fact that much surgery is without valid reason I am stating no more than has been repeatedly stated by leading members of the surgical profession itself.

On the plane of instinct this lack of desire for food is duly respected. The sick dog hides. He will not eat. He refuses a wet compress on his brow. He does not feel sorry for himself and does not seek for sympathy. He refuses to permit his friends to hold his paws.

All he wants is to be left alone. He wants no food and he takes none. Rest, quiet, warmth, air and, sometimes, a little water, are all he wants. He will not take juices or diluted milk, if offered these, nor will he take the juice of flesh. Vitamins, if proffered, will be rejected. Resting in seclusion, preferably in a dark place, while awaiting the completion of the reparative work done by his own self-healing power—he recovers.

There is order in the processes of nature; the haphazard nowhere reigns supreme. There must be, thus, some profound reason for the suspension of digestive processes and the simultaneous suspension of the desire for food in states of acute illness. The sick man's dislike of food would seem to be as significant as his dislike of noise, motion, light, close air and cold. Yet, while these latter dislikes are commonly respected, we are inclined to disregard the first and attempt to feed in spite of the most obstinate repugnance to food.

If the patient is chilly, we warm him; if noise disturbs him, we seek to protect him from this; if light disturbs him, we lower the shades; if the air is close, we open the windows; we respect his desire to lie quietly and not move about. But we urge him to eat.

There is a story told of Pope Leo XIII, that, in his last illness in his ninety-third year, he said to his physicians: "Gentlemen, you require me to eat more than I ate in health."

This practice was all too common and is still responsible for much unnecessary suffering and death. Going without food in acute disease not only relieves pain, but rests the heart and relieves the kidneys. The ancients well understood the value of abstinence in acute disease and an understanding of its value was carried down even into late times. Fasting in fevers was commonly employed by Neapolitan physicians over a hundred and fifty years ago. They frequently permitted their fever patients to go for as many as forty days without food.

It should not be thought, however, that fasting should be instituted only in states of serious illness, that one should continue to eat so long as any digestive power remains. On the contrary, missing a few meals at the beginning of the trouble is often enough to prevent the development of serious trouble. If functional impairment is only slight, as indicated by a coated tongue, headache, a general malaise, and similar "insignificant" symptoms, a short fast will enable the body to eliminate the systemic toxemia before more formidable trouble evolves.

If, when the first symptoms appear, the patient were put to bed, strict repose enjoined, no good given, many cases of acute disease would be light and of short duration. The patient should be kept warm and given all the water demanded by thirst. The room should be light and airy, and visitors should be excluded. Rest is the important thing.

When the acute sufferer fasts his discomforts are less severe, his pains are less intense, his fever does not rise so high, complications are rare, loss of weight is often less than in the patient who does not fast, and the duration of the disease shortened. Less weight loss is almost, if not entirely due to the fact that the duration of the disease is shortened. Typhoid fever, as an example, lasts in the average case from eight to twelve days instead of the usual twenty-one days. The courses of measles, scarlet fever and pneumonia are correspondingly shortened.

Again we reiterate: Fasting is not a *cure*.

But, conducted properly, the physiological rest it provides the body's organs can often help the recovery forces of nature carry out the healing work.

18

Fasting in Chronic Disease

"I have lost my appetite."

"Nothing tastes good to me any more. I eat only as a matter of routine."

"I suffer with distress after every meal."

These are some of the complaints of patients who suffer with some chronic form of disease, such as colitis, chronic gastritis, hay fever, asthma, arthritis, nervousness, stomach ulcer or cancer.

These people eat, only because they honestly think that they must eat—regularly, every day, three times a day—to stay alive. Some of them are overweight, but great numbers of them are thin and remain so, although they may be overeating.

Another class of chronic sufferers are, as they put it, "always hungry."

They eat at all hours of the day and night. They habitually overeat, whipping up their jaded sense of taste with condiments, strong flavors, and in other ways. Often they suffer after each meal but they don't cut down on their intake. Then there are those among this class who suffer almost as much when they do not eat as when they do.

"Hunger" here, as we have seen in other cases, is not hunger at all, in a true sense, but a morbid sensation or set of sensations mistaken for hunger. It may be a "gnawing" in the stomach, pain in the stomach or some other symptom of gastric irritation. This is the reason the sensation cannot be satisfied. The fact that eating palliates the discomfort for a few moments, does not prove that food was actually needed, any more than the need for a cup of coffee is proven when it temporarily relieves a coffee addict's headache. The surest, simplest way for those who are "always hungry" to overcome their supposed hunger is to fast.

Man tends to abstain from food when under great emotional distress. Rejection of food is frequent among the insane. Although it is the present practice to use force to feed mentally ill patients, it is doubtful if such enforced feeding is proper. Man instinctively fasts under certain conditions, as do the lower animals, and the rejection of food by the mentally ill is probably an instinctive act that will, if not interrupted, prove very beneficial. Indeed, my experience with such patients has convinced me that this is true.

The most important feature about fasting in chronic disease is the marked acceleration of elimination that it occasions, thus speedily freeing the body of its accumulated toxic load. The disappearance of symptoms, sometimes of years standing, when one fasts, is often dramatic. Fasting provides opportunity for the body to do for itself what it is unable to do under conditions of surfeit. Surfeit makes impossible the cleaning of the fluids and tissues in a physiological housecleaning.

A properly conducted fast will enable the chronically ill body to excrete the toxic load that is responsible for the trouble, after which a corrected mode of living enables the individual to evolve into a vigorous state of health.

It should not be thought that eating must be continued so long as the body does not vigorously rebel against food. When there is functional impairment, symptoms of impairment, sluggishness and unease, then is the time to institute what may be described as a *preventive fast*. A fast at this point need not be long. Improvement often is swift—preventing an evolution of serious sickness. When we observe the eyes become brighter, the skin fairer, and the breath sweeter while fasting, or when we see a poor complexion clear up, or other symptoms fade and vigor return—we can be certain that the fast has enabled the body to carry out a preventive housecleaning.

It is a mistake to expect one fast, even a long one, to be sufficient to enable the body to free itself of the whole of its accumulated debris. A lifetime of piling up toxins cannot be corrected in the span of a few weeks. In such diseases as paralysis agitans, arthritis, a large tumor, and other conditions that require so much time to build, three or more fasts are often needed to obtain all the improvement possible in a particular case.

Sinusitis is inflammation of the nasal sinuses. It would have been called a catarrhal condition by our fathers and mothers, but the tendency today is to discontinue the use of a general term like catarrh and to use so-called specific terms. Sinusitis may be either acute or chronic. Most people have some inflammation in one of more parts of the mucous membranes of the body—that is to say, they have one or more "catarrhs."

Names of *catarrhal inflammations* vary with the different locations, but it is all the same disease with the same general cause. The practice of classifying each local inflammation by a different name and giving each an individuality, confuses both the patient and the physician. This keeps alive the delusion that there are many *diseases*.

Replying to the charge that fasting lowers resistance to disease, Dr. Weger says: "I have seen many cases of infection of different kinds recover completely on a fast. Take for example an advanced case of sinusitis after five or six painful operations—frontal, ethmoidal, and antrum—with surgical drainage and irrigations two or three times a week, continued over a period of two to five years, with no relief or amelioration of symptoms. After almost unendurable suffering, such patients are as a rule, thin, and physically and mentally depressed. When they make complete recoveries after a prolonged fast, as the great majority of them do, is this not sufficient proof that fasting somehow or other raises the power of the organism to overcome infection, rather than fasting renders them more susceptible? What is true of sinusitis is equally true of other infections—even those so situated anatomically that they cannot be surgically drained, and must therefore be absorbed."

What is here said of recovery from sinusitis is equally true of recovery from other inflammations in the respiratory, digestive, genitourinary tracts and other regions of the body that are lined with mucous membrane.

Thus otitis, conjunctivitis, gastritis, duodenitis, ileitis, colitis, metritis—all have been known to clear up during the course of a lengthy fast. Only in comparatively rare instances are two fasts required. Hay fever and asthma, both belonging to this same group of "diseases," are remedied by the forces of the organism during a fast.

Extensive experience with fasting in a wide variety of diseases, running over a period of more than a hundred and thirty years and involving the work of hundreds of men and women caring for many thousands of patients, has demonstrated that when the load is lifted from the digestive organs by fasting, all of the energy of the body is transferred to the organs of excretion, permitting full use of these organs in freeing the body of an accumulated load of toxin.

What the body can do for itself in the way of restoring normal function and full vigor when the toxic load is lifted has to be seen to be fully appreciated.

Speaking of pernicious anemia, Tilden says: "A fast of two weeks, without anything at all except water, will improve anemia condition by increasing the blood-corpuscles sometimes by five hundred thousand in that length of time." There is poisoning from the digestive tract in all of these cases and it seems most likely that this befoulment of the blood with sepsis from this source is the cause of the failure of the blood-making organs.

A similar septic befoulment seems to exist in cancer, causing anemia in this condition. It should be emphasized strongly that no person suffering with anemia should undertake a fast, except under competent supervision.

There is an equal need for experienced supervision of the diabetic who fasts. The diabetic may safely and profitably fast, particularly if he carries considerable weight. If insulin has been taken over an extended period of time, fasting is rarely recommended.

The sufferer with Bright's disease may also fast with great benefit. In both these conditions and all similar "diseases," more important than the fast is the correction of the total way of life. It is imperative that these patients be taught how to eat and that they learn their individual limitations and to respect these. They may evolve into good health—continually improved health—if all enervating habits are discontinued and the patient learns the laws of proper eating.

19

The Case of the Common Cold

Millions of dollars have been spent in trying to discover what germ or set of germs produces the common cold. All the efforts so far have led on to greater confusion, greater claims and greater expenditures on remedies and the quest for vaccines to prevent colds.

Harold Deihs, M.D., at the University of Minnesota, tested, on many thousands of students, virtually every cold remedy ever devised and kept exact records. None of them proved to be a genuine remedy.

Some authorities insist that the cold is caused by a whole panoply of cold microbes—a sort of "germ cocktail." Other common cold experts propound the concept that the cold is produced by a virus or a whole series of viruses. Nearly a hundred viruses have been identified which may play some role in the causation of the cold. As all work now seems to be concentrated on finding a vaccine that will *immunize* one against these viruses, it is obvious that a number of vaccines will have to be perfected. It would be so much better to learn to live in a manner to avoid colds. The normal body produces its own protection. It needs no outside crutch.

It has been said that the cold is common, not because it is simple, but because it is so complex. This may have reference to the confusion in which the etiology of the cold has been enshrouded. Dr. Tilden said that a cold is the proximal symptom of a complex whose distal symptom is cancer or tuberculosis or some other fatal *degenerative disease*.

Between the first cold of infancy and death from cancer in middle life, there are intermediate complexes and symptoms galore—colds, coughs, sore throats, constipation, diarrhea, headaches, fatigue, grouchiness, apprehension, restlessness, sleeplessness, bad breath, coated tongue, and many other symptoms and so-called acute diseases, all of which are but crises in toxemia. The non-toxemic individual cannot be made to develop symptoms of a cold.

In humorous verse, but with underlying truth, the *rationale* of the causes of cold was presented in these stanzas in a poem published in the *American Journal of Clinical Medicine* in 1928:

> A cold is not a cold to me—
>   It's Nature's way to tell
> That I've been dining recently
>   Not wisely, but too well.
>
> A snuffy nose has come to mean
>   That I've enjoyed erstwhile
> Some breaded porkchops, nested deep
>   In sweet spuds, southern style. . . .
>
> Or else, perchance, a wondrous steak,
>   With onions crisp and brown,
> Has made my liver make of me
>   A menace to the town.
>
> Or, it might be a chunk of cheese,
>   Or mince pie hot and sweet,
> So, a cold is not a cold to me—
>   It's just too much to eat.

Hygienists can fully endorse the thoughts expressed in these lines. Not only may one avoid colds by learning to eat within limitations and by conserving energy in every way, but one may hasten the termination of the cold by fasting. Stuffing the patient who has a cold is a sure way of prolonging it and of causing it to "run into pneumonia" or something else. Few people realize the importance of stopping all food until all symptoms have subsided.

In an article on the common cold, published in American newspapers on Dec. 20, 1962, Dr. Walter C. Alvarez, professor of medicine and editor of *American Medicine*, and newspaper columnist, declared: "In the great British cold research laboratory at Salisbury, it was found that sitting or standing in wet clothes in a draft does not produce a cold."

Such experiments are but wasteful repetitions of experiments that were conducted in this country in the last century by *Hygienists*, and, while they confirm the conclusions arrived at by the *Hygienists*, they add nothing new to our knowledge of the cause of colds. Alvarez says that he himself has no fear of getting chilled in winter.

Alvarez thinks that colds are "contagious." He says that what he does fear is to get into a taxi cab with a man who has a sniffy cold. He thinks that he "catches cold" or what it catches him under such circumstances. As such an experience never causes me to have a cold, I wonder why he so readily develops a cold when thus "exposed." He discounts the idea that being in good condition will enable one to avoid colds, but his reasons for objecting to this idea are rather shaky.

In his youth he used to have four severe colds a year—at a time when he was an athlete, a track man, a swimmer and an instructor in a gymnasium—although he would take a cold bath every morning and run three or four miles every evening.

Unfortunately for his position, his activities do not necessarily prove that he was in genuinely good condition. Athletes are notorious for their frequent colds. Alvarez has accepted the common faulty conception of what constitutes good condition. A plethoric and toxemic individual may pass for being in good condition. He says: "We are told to eat well and get plenty of sleep." He neither approves nor disapproves of this advice. I would point out that what is commonly meant by "eating well" is overeating and eating plentifully of staple foods. This is a sure way to build colds, not to prevent them.

I do not dismiss exposure to cold, however, as a contributing factor in the production of a cold any more than I am willing to dismiss becoming overheated as a contributing factor in the same complex of factors that collectively constitute cause. Prolonged exposure to cold enervates and this checks elimination.

Those who are already enervated and toxemic, when exposed to cold, have their elimination further checked and this is frequently enough to precipitate a crisis, in this case a cold. It should be realized that when one is already enervated and toxemic any added enervating influence will place enough additional check upon elimination that a crisis is sure to develop.

What happens is that the added check upon elimination causes the toxic accumulation to rise above the point of established toleration and the body rebels. A channel of supplementary elimination is established through which to get rid of the excess.

Copavin, the drug considered the best by Alvarez, was the only one that Diehs thought "worked well." This drug, which contains codeine, was said to "block out" about 85% of colds, but it was "effective" only if taken early. It does not *cure* the cold later. The fact is that the many "block outs" attributed to this drug would have occurred had the drug not been given. Colds last anywhere from a few hours to two or three weeks. Almost anything can be made to appear to *cure* the cold for the reason that recovery is spontaneous and occurs if nothing is done. *Copavin* results in constipation and troubles many nervous patients. It does not remove the cause of the cold.

What should we do when the first symptom of a cold arises? All food should be discontinued at once. Instead of large quantities of water, as commonly advised, only as much water as thirst demands should be taken. Indeed, it seems that the less water taken the more rapid the recovery. The fast should not be less than twenty-four hours, it may be three or four days in duration, depending on the severity of the symptoms.

Following the fast, eating should be light for the first few days: orange or a grapefruit—no sugar—for breakfast, a vegetable salad at noon, and fresh fruit in season in the evening, for the first one to two days, after which the eating should be sparse until all symptoms have subsided.

While fasting, the best place for the patient is in bed. He should be warm and comfortable and should have fresh air in the room both day and night. A daily lukewarm bath may be taken, but no heroic bathing is advisable. If it is not possible to quit work and go to bed, one should obtain as much rest as circumstances permit and get to bed early at night.

If these simple suggestions are carried out, no cold will evolve into pneumonia. Prolonging a cold by eating and by suppressing its symptoms with drugs, may end in death.

Fasting does not *cure* a cold. One may get well of a cold if one eats heartily, drinks heavily, gets little sleep, works hard and is chilled by day. People have been doing this throughout history. All that we claim for the foregoing fasting program is that it greatly lessens the discomforts of the cold, shortens its duration and leaves the patient in much better condition when the cold has ended.

20

Multiple Sclerosis

Widespread fund-raising campaigns to fight the crippling effects of this disease, and to perform research into its cause and treatment, have made multiple sclerosis familiar to the public. Yet there may be some basic causes already known in terms of diet and activities of the individual and even possible avenues of recovery in the fast.

I recall a case of an optometrist whose condition became so bad that he had to give up his work and turn his office over to someone else. For a few years he had been under the care of several of the best neurologists of the East and, as they had warned him at the outset, had grown progressively worse. They had frankly told him that they had no *cure* for multiple sclerosis.

They were telling him the truth, yet after seven weeks in a *Hygienic* institution, he walked out under his own power, returned home and resumed his professional activities.

He was not a well man at the end of seven weeks. It is too much to expect a full recovery in such a short time. But he had made such great improvement that he felt justified in returning home and getting back to work. This is often a wrong position to take, especially with a condition like multiple sclerosis, but it is a mistake that the sick frequently make.

Many patients seem to be satisfied to stop their efforts in recovering health when they have been freed of their most annoying symptoms. They are often unwilling to go on to full health, and are convinced they can take care of themselves. After having made a certain amount of initial improvement they expect to take charge and they feel they can carry on, from that point, as well as their professional adviser. In a few cases it works out; generally they fail. In cases watched and controlled, results of fasting can be established.

Sclerosis means induration or hardening. It has special reference to hardening of a part due to inflammation. In the nervous system the term denotes an overgrowth of connective tissue (hyperplasia of connective tissue) in the nerve tissue.

Multiple sclerosis—also called disseminated sclerosis and sometimes

99

known as Charcot's disease—is characterized by hardening (sclerosis) occurring in sporadic patches through the brain and spinal cord or both. These hardened patches range from the size of a pin head to that of a pea and are scattered irregularly through the brain and cord.

At autopsy, it is found that the insulating sheath of the nerves is broken down and the nerve cells and fibers have fused together. I have emphasized that this is what is found at autopsy for the reason that the trouble does not start as a sclerosis (hardening), but as an inflammation.

A man dies after suffering with multiple sclerosis for fifteen or twenty years and an autopsy is performed. His brain and nervous system are subjected to the closest scrutiny and certain pathological changes are found. But this is the end-point. What was the condition of his nerves five years, ten years or fifteen years prior to death? It is reasonable to think that if the condition of the nerves was the same five years or ten years prior to death that they are found to be in at death, he would have died five to ten years earlier.

The disease is said to be "incurable." It may last for years before the patient dies. The end-point, as found at death, is certainly irreversible, but can we be sure that the earlier stages of the disease are irreversible? The very progress of the disease would seem to negate such an assumption. In the inflammatory stage of the disease it would certainly seem to be remediable.

Indeed, spontaneous remissions are known that may last for weeks or even years. Once the hardening has occurred, there would seem to be no possibility that the disease could intermit, or that recovery could be effected.

A fatty insulating material called the myelin sheath, which surrounds the nerves, is lost and this is said to cause abnormal nerve behavior. Some of the nerves work energetically, some work very weakly and others fail to work at all.

No two cases are alike because in no two cases are the same parts of the brain and nervous system affected. The development of the hardening does not progress at the same rate in each case, and does not take place at the same rate at all points in the body of the same patient. For the reason that no two cases are identical, no description of the disease will fit any particular case.

Among the leading symptoms of the disease are weakness, strong jerky movements, incoordination of the extremities that is often more marked in the arms than in the legs, and amemomania, which is a form of insanity with agreeable hallucinations. Also other abnormal mental exaltations, scanning speech and an involuntary rapid movement of the eyes, called nyastagmus are evident. The tremor is jerky, is increased by voluntary efforts to restrain it, and is entirely absent during complete rest and sleep, returning when movements are resumed.

The nature of the symptoms in each case will depend on the locations and severity of the changes in the nervous tissues. A sudden loss of vision in one eye or a period of double vision may be an early symptom. The eye symptoms usually clear up in a short time and they may not recur for months or years. The patient may develop peculiar feelings, with tingling and numbness in various parts of the limbs and body.

Weakness in the legs and difficulty in walking may later develop. There may be trembling, jerking of the legs, difficulty in talking, a hand may become clumsy or useless. Tremor of the hand may develop when the individual attempts to pick up something. Trouble with the rectum and the urinary bladder may also develop.

These symptoms may remain mild for a number of years or they may clear up and not recur for long periods. It is this remission of symptoms that indicates that in the early stages of the disease the developments are not irreversible. About half of these patients are still able to work after twenty-five years, a fact which indicates the slowness of the development of the disease. This certainly provides ample time for something constructive to be done.

Many cases are so mild and the symptoms so evanescent that they are not diagnosed as sclerosis for years. The tendency of the symptoms to cease for periods of time is said to be one of the basic characteristics of the disease, the other being the scattered character of the symptomatic developments, as the hardening is scattered.

I have previously pointed out that no two cases are alike in their symptoms or in their development, each patient lending his own individuality to the disease; but this is no more true of multiple sclerosis than of any other disease.

No germ or virus has been found upon which to lay the blame for the development of the disease and it is freely confessed that "the cause is unknown." It is, however, thought to be "probably of infectious origin."

No treatment has proved satisfactory. This is true in so many diseases that it is almost the rule. How can there be satisfactory treatment of a disease the cause of which is unrecognized? Standard works on the disease say: "The cause of the disease is entirely unknown . . . there is no specific or really effective treatment . . . always a long-standing disease, total recovery from it is very doubtful."

Certainly we cannot expect total recovery if the cause is unrecognized. The failure to recognize the general impairing influences in the life and environment of the patient as the true cause of functional and organic deterioration blinds us to the causes of disease.

The search for specific causes has about reached its end. The time has arrived when we must find in wrong living habits the cause of the failures of the organism and the evolution of its diseases. When these are recognized and removed, there is a possibility of recovery in thousands of individuals who are now regarded as hopelessly *incurable*.

I have never had opportunity to care for a case of multiple sclerosis in the early stages, hence I can only suggest that if these cases were given *Hygienic* care at the outset of their trouble, the percentage of recoveries would be high. All of the cases I have had the privilege of caring for have been in advanced stages and I do not consider these favorable cases.

The fact that I have been able to return some of these, even in helpless conditions, to a state of usefulness speaks volumes for the efficiency of the *Hygienic* program in restoring normal tissue and functional condition.

Let us review the general picture of the fasting experience, as applied to a multiple sclerosis case. The first fast brings about remarkable improvement in the general health of the individual with considerable increase in his control and use of his limbs, often enabling the bed-ridden patient to get up and walk about. He manages to hold this improvement and not infrequently to add to it, while eating a carefully planned diet and taking regular exercise and sun baths following the fast.

A second fast adds to his control and use of his limbs. I have employed as many as three fasts in these cases. Each fast has resulted in increased control of the limbs and has made it possible for them to be used with greater ease.

I continue the rest in bed following the fast, adding a period or two of daily light exercise of a type that requires increasing skill in their performance. The purpose of the exercise in these cases is not so much that of increasing the size and strength of the muscles as to increase the individual's skill in their use. Heavier exercise may come later if desired.

I am convinced that daily sunbathing in these cases is especially helpful in furthering the evolution of nerve health. The diet is one of fresh fruits and vegetables with only moderate quantities of fats, sugars, starches and proteins. I prefer the vegetable proteins—nuts and sunflower seeds are good in these cases.

The important thing for us to remember is that the sclerosis does not belong to the initial stages of the disease. In these early stages recovery is most likely to take place, providing only that all impairing influences are removed from the life of the individual and his blood and flesh are freed of their toxic load.

It is in the initial stage that full recovery is or should be possible, not in the advanced stages when irreversible changes in the nerve structures have taken place. The ancient adage: "A stitch in time"—in this case, action in time, can make the difference.

21

Asthma

A young soprano whose voice and hard work had won her the high honor of being a member of the Metropolitan Opera found herself in a heartbreaking situation: She had developed a serious asthmatic condition and could no longer sing.

Her physician told her frankly, "I can give you temporary respite. We have no cure for asthma."

The desperate singer consulted a specialist who reiterated what the family physician had told her. There was no *cure*.

At that moment this singer faced the prospect of the wreckage of her career, in spite of her talent, training, work and dreams. She gave up singing. She retired to her farm in New Jersey. Medicine had written off her chances.

Then she heard of *Natural Hygiene*—the concept of the importance of the body's own healing capacity. Uncertain—but willing in her predicament to try any possible avenue of help, she consulted a *Hygienist*.

After examining her and hearing her story, he told her, "You can be helped. I believe you can free yourself of this asthmatic condition if you will do what I tell you—not by medicine or medical treatment at all."

"What then?" she demanded.

"Simply fast."

She did not understand. He explained at length to her the processes of fasting as we have been discussing them and their techniques in this book.

The young singer grasped at this idea that was entirely new and startling to her.

The fast did the job.

In a matter not of months but of weeks the asthma cleared, within a few months she was back at the Metropolitan. A career that might otherwise have been smashed on the rocks of asthmatic suffering was able to return to its triumphant course.

In both the United States and Canada today are thousands of men and women of all ages who have recovered without any attention being given to the things to which they were told they were allergic.

Indeed, as I have so often stressed, once they have been restored to full health, they can take a bath in pollens of all kinds without any ill effects. I have seen long lists of the foods and other substances to which patients have been shown by the scratch test to be *allergic*.

An asthmatic undergoing a fast was in my office one morning when a cat walked into the room. The asthmatic looked startled—then laughed. "Before coming here," he told me, "I would have had an attack of asthma if a cat walked into a room where I happened to be." He picked up the cat, held it in his arms, and proceeded to stroke its back. "It feels good to be able to breathe again."

He had been sent from New England to Arizona, where five years of the "climate *cure*" had done him no appreciable good. Asthmatics suffer year after year, often becoming worse with the passage of time, when all of them could get well in four to eight weeks and remain well for the remainder of their lives.

Standard text books name several varieties of asthma—including cardiac, renal and bronchial, and describe many complications. As we regard all varieties of asthma and all so-called complications as symptoms rising out of the same general cause, and requiring the same general corrections of the mode of living, we may ignore, for the present, these differentiations. The symptom-complexes that are named different disease require special attention only in so far as it is needful to know where possible, if organic change is so great as to make recovery impossible.

We must not forget the unity of disease and the unity of cause that binds all the so-called diseases together. The different so-called diseases get their names from the tissues and organs involved in the pathological process. The symptoms are characteristic of the organs and tissues and not of the poisoning.

Renal asthma is seen in advanced kidney disease and cardiac asthma is seen in severe heart disease. In both instances the difficult breathing is due to an accumulation of fluid in the lungs and to other changes in the lungs. Recovery from these types of asthma depends upon recovery from the heart or kidney disease. As asthma in these diseases is a development in the late stages, recovery is not always possible.

Bronchial asthma, which is defined as recurrent paroxysms of difficult breathing (dyspnea) and coughing, is a catarrhal condition involving the mucous membrane of the lower respiratory passages. The asthma is more or less spasmodic and is always accompanied by catarrhal affections in other parts of the body. There is a catarrh of the nose and throat, commonly sinusitis, often gastritis or colitis and metritis or cystitis. Indeed, the catarrh exists for some time before asthmatic symptoms appear.

Asthma is found everywhere, in all classes of peple. It is found in both warm and cold countries, in wet and dry climates, in high and low altitudes, among the rich and in the poor, the high and the low, the short and thin, the fat and the lean, the light and the dark. Men, women and children develop the disease and it is seen at times in pampered animals. In those very climates to which asthmatics are sometimes sent to seek a *cure*, people native to the community and the climate often develop asthma.

Two people practice bad habits for years, one of them being about as indulgent as the other, and one of them develops asthma, the other develops arthritis. Why does one pay for his bad habits in one way and the other in another? We are in the habit of saying that this is due to diathesis or predisposition, but these are words that explain little.

Why is one so disposed and the other differently disposed? Why does one man develop kidney disease and another man develop gallstones? Why do two men equally exposed to the rigors of a blizzard not both develop pneumonia? Why does one have pneumonia and the other only a cold? Why does one man have bronchial catarrh for years and never develop asthmatic symptoms, and another have the same catarrh and also the asthmatic symptoms? It is now customary to say that one is allergic and the other is not, but this is another word that explains nothing.

The asthmatic is a neurotic; by this, I mean that he is predisposed to develop nervous diseases. But what is the predisposition? The answer, I believe firmly, lies primarily in constitutional weaknesses, growing, in many instances, out of heredity, in other cases out of larval deficiencies, resulting from faulty nutrition in the parents and grandparents.

Other factors that may be involved in producing what is called predisposition are habit and environmental stresses. Tobacco stresses the heart and lungs overeating stresses the liver and kidneys; too much physical activity stresses the heart and joints; fear stresses the heart and nervous system. These are but samples of stresses to organs and systems that are part of the conventional ways of life. Such stresses weaken and impair organs and functions and lay the groundwork for local pathological evolutions.

Cold and heat and dryness and wetness and other environmental factors may place enough stress upon the body to do harm. Sudden extremes of such factors may precipitate a crisis.

We trace asthma, as we do all other so-called diseases, to a blood and flesh condition which we denominate toxemia. It is caused by a mode of living that expends nerve energy excessively, brings on a state of nerve fatigue which we call enervation, so that the functions of life are carried on at a low physiological level. Consequently, elimination of waste is checked so that it tends to accumulate in the blood, lymph and tissues.

The presence of more than a physiological amount of waste in the body—at all times there is waste being carried by the blood and lymph away from the cells for excretion—results in irritation and inflammation. In those individuals in whom this development takes place, the foundation for asthma is laid in the respiratory tract.

That this explanation of the cause of asthma is valid is shown by the fact that elimination of toxemia, restoration of normal nerve energy and correction of the mode of living results in a permanent clearing up of symptoms and the individual no longer suffers with asthma. As no other means of care results in a more rapid freeing of the body of its toxic load than physiological rest, nothing brings relief from asthmatic paroxysms as certainly and as speedily as the fast.

But relief is not all the sufferer wishes. He wants to get well and this is precisely what he accomplishes if the fast is conducted long enough and his mode of eating and living after the fast are made to conform to his genuine physiological needs.

The length of the fast required to enable the asthmatic to breathe freely and easily will depend on the severity of the condition. Usually within twenty-four to thirty-six hours the worst cases are enabled to lie flat in their beds and to breathe easily and sleep. Breathing is not normal at this stage, as the stethoscope quickly reveals. There will be rales in the lungs, as there will be mucus in these structures. Indeed, the secretion of mucus will not cease for several days.

I favor carrying the fast to the clearing up of all abnormal sounds in the lungs, if this is possible. In very thin and weak individuals this is not always to be recommended. In such instances, a fast as long as it is safe must be followed by a period of light eating and then another fast is recommended. In long-standing cases of this kind, several short fasts and periods of careful feeding may be required before full recovery results.

Some fasting advocates advise not taking nourishment until at least thirty-six hours after all asthmatic symptoms have cleared up. But these experts also urge a return to the fast if eating is followed by asthmatic sensations. The recurrence of symptoms so soon after eating is resumed is certain evidence that the fast has not been carried far enough to permit full systematic readjustment.

I do not favor playing with asthma in this manner. In the long run, where a more extended fast is possible, it will prove more effective and the results will be far more satisfactory.

22

Arthritis: Two Years or Twenty-eight?

"Two years!" exclaimed a patient, when told it would require a minimum of two years for him to get well of his arthritis by fasting and other *Hygienic* methods. "I have taken twenty-eight years already. What are two more years?"

He had been a bacteriologist working in a laboratory and giving nothing more than the usual attention to his health, when he developed the first signs of arthritis. He was in intimate daily contact with physicians of the highest order and received the best care the profession had to offer in this disease. But, as is generally known and is admitted by the profession, no cure for the disease exists. Palliation—relieving symptoms without removing the cause of the disease—is all that is provided, and this does not prevent the spread and intensification of the trouble.

With the passage of the years, joint after joint became involved until, when the foregoing remark was made to a *Hygienist* who had been consulted, the patient was a twisted and distorted man walking with the aid of crutch and cane, in a much stooped position. He was unable to turn his head from side to side, and in constant pain.

He was told that there was a possibility that some of his joints were ankylosed—fused—and that, if so, these joints would remain ankylosed. There is no way to un-fuse ankylosed joints. They remain fixed, immovable. The good news was, in this case, however, that he could be freed of pain. He could be restored to usefulness and he could enjoy life.

This man underwent a lengthy fast—one of thirty-six days. There was great improvement. He was freed of pain, witnessed the disappearance of swelling from some of his joints, its reduction in others and the slow return of movement to joints that had long been stiff.

Two years were not enough. It took four years to complete all the improvement possible in this man. During this time he had a second long fast and several fasts of a few days each. His eating between fasts was carefully supervised; he was given daily sun baths and after a certain amount of initial improvement had been made, he was given daily exercise.

Result: his spine is almost straight, the use of his arms and legs is normal, he can turn his head, he walks in a nearly upright position, he does not use cane or crutch, he has no pain, he looks the "picture of health," and he works like a slave.

He has remained in excellent health with no recurrence of pain or swelling for a period of seven years, and feels so well that he has taken on a lot of political activities in addition to his regular work, which is enough for one man.

His was an extreme case and required a lengthy period for recovery. Let us consider for contrast a milder case, of shorter duration with less joint inflammation and stiffness: Mrs. G. was forty-four years old. She was the wife of a Canadian school principal. Her arthritis was of but a few months standing, but it was painful and crippled her movements. Mrs. G's physician could promise her nothing but temporary relief which was aspirin or cortisone for the rest of her life. He told her there would be a probable spreading and increase of pain. She journeyed to the States and underwent a fast. The fast lasted only three weeks, but it freed her of all pain and inflammation and restored normal movement to her joints.

"I am going to advertise you all over Canada," she said to the *Hygienist* who conducted her fast and after-care. She kept her word, but the important thing in this connection is that, after the passage of over three years, she is still free of arthritis. She has had no recurrence of pain and inflammation. Her enthusiasm for fasting in particular and *Hygiene* in general knows no bounds.

These two cases may be taken as typical of hundreds of similar cases the writer has seen recover during the past more than forty years. Not all of these recoveries have continued on for years without recurrence; some of the individuals were foolish enough to return to their former disease-producing mode of living, but they have been able to remedy the recurrences by returning to good physical behavior, so that they have remained well.

Keeping well requires that we give a reasonable amount of intelligent attention to the manner in which we live. It takes no more time and effort to eat sensibly than it does to eat imprudently and indiscriminately. One must breathe—it requires no more time to breathe pure air than it does to breathe impure air. Indeed, in all the ways of living, not more time, often less time is required to live rightly than wrongly.

Why shall we go through life taking an antacid after each meal, when it is possible to eat in such a way that we can at all times be comfortable after meals? Why shall we take aspirin for recurrent headaches, when we can live in a manner to avoid headaches? Why take a daily laxative, when it is easily possible to have normal bowel movements? The intelligent reader will have no difficulty in answering these questions.

Discomfort has meaning to the observing and reasoning individual. The intelligent man should see in all discomforts and pains hints of warnings that he should slow down and eliminate some of his indulgences. He should heed their warnings. Nature is a remarkable teacher and if we accept her instructions and observe her warning signs, health and long life will be ours.

Because of its very painful nature and its tendency to completely incapacitate the sufferer, rheumatic arthritis is one of the most serious and most dreaded disease of man. Developing, as it does in the joints, it soon, unless its causes are removed, makes an invalid or a semi-invalid of the patient. The pain is so severe and so persistent that it rapidly destroys all peace of mind and prevents rest and sleep. Although probably developing most frequently in cold, damp areas, arthritis is found in all localities.

Several varieties of arthritis are known, but listing then is of no practical importance. Were we laboriously to draw a picture of each of the several varities in the forms of the disease, we would be but filling up space and wearying the reader. All of these several variations are traceable to the same underlying cause, and are remediable by eliminating this cause.

Pain and swelling of the tissues surrounding the joints are prominent features of the early stages of arthritis. As soon as inflammation develops, efforts are made to immobilize the joint. The muscles and ligaments become tensed and contracted, the on-guard condition thus developed seemingly increasing the pain.

Involving as it does the joints, especially the surrounding tissues, arthritis presents a more complicated problem than the more simple, transient pains and aches that may be called rheumatism, such as lumbago, or so-called muscular rheumatism. Developing, as it frequently does, in the cartilage that pads the ends of the bones of the joints, the arthritis may lead to destruction of the cartilage and produce deformity.

If the cause is not removed, the denuded ends of the bones will ultimately unite (ankylose) so that the joint becomes fixed and immovable. When this bony union takes place the pain ceases, but the joint is forever lost.

Rheumatic arthritis is not built in a day. The vigorous and strong may practice enervating habits for years before it evolves. Or such individuals may, after its first appearance, hold it in check for years before it becomes a serious crippling influence. We should know that arthritis represents an end-point in a pathological process that has been years in its development.

Before the development of the joint inflammation, there are aches and pains, with periods of not feeling well, periods of not being able to sleep, of poor appetite, of indigestion, and of other evidences that all is not well within. So long as we continue to close our eyes to the existence of the many "minor" symptoms and refuse to recognize them as forerunners of the more complex stages of disease, just so long will we refuse to make those changes in our way of life that are essential to the prevention of arthritis.

How often do people who are bothered with vague musuclar pains, a little stiffening of the joints, a "touch of neuritis," an "attack" of lumbago or of sciatica, mistake the significance of these warning signs. They palliate these symptoms with drugs, massage, manipulations, hot baths, and persist in the way of life that builds trouble.

Suppressing symptoms does nothing to remove their causes and fails to check the further development of a chronic state and the possible development of invalidism.

Fundamentally and primarily the cause of arthritis is toxemia. This is the summing up of a multitude of abuses of the body in eating, drinking, emoting, in sexual activity, and in other forms of activity. Eating too much from childhood lays the foundation for the toxemia. No one knows just how many subtle toxins are involved in the cause of arthritis. It may be said that hundreds or even thousands may be involved in its production.

Years will elapse before it becomes possible to isolate all the compounds amino acids alone are capable of forming with one another and with other by-products of proteins and carbohydrates. It is safe to assume that no single poison is alone and independently responsible for the evolution of any complex pathology.

How can we hope, in our present state of ignorance, to isolate and analyze one particular toxic substance that is the cause of cancer or of Bright's disease or of insanity? Can it be asserted with any degree of assurance that the toxins responsible for any one or all of the so-called degenerative diseases differ in any essential? The character of the disease resulting from the toxic saturation is determined by individual factors rather than by the character of the toxin.

I describe the cause of arthritis as a perversion of nutrition in a toxemic subject. There seems to be no doubt that the primary irritation leading to the abnormal changes in the joints is due to the presence in the blood and lymph of an unstable toxic material accumulating for months and years in one who is enervated. These sufferers are always heavy eaters, but are especially prone to overeat on sweets and starches—bread, potatoes, cakes, pies and candy.

Their joints are likely to be stiff and they find it difficult to get around in the morning when they first arise. Stiffness wears off after a little use of the limbs, but the knee joints, ankle joints, elbow joints, and other joints of the body are likely to complain bitterly when used. There may be no pain and there are rarely any constitutional symptoms, so that the patient is likely to think that the stiffness is entirely local.

Wrong food combinations, excesses of starches and sugars, condiments, coffee, tea, liquors, and tobacco are potent factors in laying the groundwork for the evolution of arthritis. Added to these factors may be any form of enervating emotional unrest, sensual indulgence, and physical overactivity. With all of this said, arthritis seems to develop only in those of the so-called gouty or arthritic or rheumatic diathesis—or predisposition. Diathesis is only a word and will remain more or less meaningless unless we understand the factors behind the predisposition.

Rheumatic arthritis, as distinguished from traumatic and tubercular arthritis, represents an impaired state of nutrition in addition to the common toxemia. The calcium deposits and stone formation that are part of the disease indicate that the nutritional perversion is similar to, if not identical with, that which is back of the formation of gall stones, kidney stones, hardening of the arteries, deposits of lime on the valves of the heart, deposits in the feet in gout, and the formation of stones in other parts of the body.

When enervation and toxemia have lowered resistance, anything that puts an added strain upon the body may precipitate an arthritic crisis in one who is predisposed to the development of arthritis. Acute illness, "infection," a "focus on infection," indigestion, an unusual meal, cold, getting wet, anxiety and overindulgence of the emotions, may precipitate a crisis.

So-called infections from abscessed teeth or abscesses elsewhere in the body should be recognized for what they are—*secondary sources of trouble*. Super-added to toxemia and gastrointestinal putrefaction, they complicate the condition of the patient. They are never primary causes.

Yet, it sometimes happens that a patient is able to resist the other sources of troubles but not these plus the secondary "infection," so that, when the source of secondary "infection" is removed, the symptoms temporarily clear up. This is heralded as a great victory for *science*. Recurrence too frequently vitiates the victory.

There have been so many kinds of treatment for arthritis that it would be needless to try to enumerate all of them. It can only be said that none of them have proved satisfactory. Spas, springs, water cures, mud, salt, soap baths, sulphur baths, hot baths, electro-therapy, packs, drugs, nostrums, and serums have all had their day and have been found wanting. Some of them have afforded temporary relief in many instances; none has been more than a palliative.

To get well and remain well of rheumatism, lumbago, muscular rheumatism, inflammatory rheumatism, gout, arthritis, no matter what form it may assume, the sufferer must discontinue all enervating habits and learn his limitations and respect them. Every normal habit indulged to satiety and every abnormal habit produces disease. Here is the origin of every so-called disease. The end is chronic disease and premature death.

Until we learn to recognize the fact that symptoms are the result of toxic saturation and learn the source of the intoxication, we are left with nothing we can do for the sick except provide a brief and questionable palliation. The man who can offer his patient nothing more than an *anodyne* or a *sedative* can do much harm but he can do no good.

To be truly effective the care of the arthritic case should be directed at the removal of the cause of the disease. To give drugs, whether aspirin, cortisone or other of the drugs now in use for arthritis, which are intended to do nothing more than provide the patient with brief periods of relief from pain, is to remove no cause. Although most of these drugs are given to "relieve" the pain, it is asserted that cortisone temporarily relieves some of the other symptoms, but it does not go beyond palliation, while it does build a more difficult condition to remedy.

The body has remarkable recuperative powers and it often succeeds in restoring health in spite of the remedies. It can do a much better and more speedy job if the remedies and the causes that have built the disease are removed. The body must be given an opportunity to eliminate its toxic accumulation by means of a fast and then an opportunity to alter its blood chemistry by means of a more or less radical change in the plan of eating. This done, the results will be surprising.

We do not restore normal nutrition by removing the effects of impaired nutrition. The proposal to cut into the arthritic joints and scrape away the deposits of lime is but a proposal to try another means of spectacular palliation. Even if it could be successfully done, it would be but a short time until more deposits would take the place of those scraped away. The cutting and the scraping would have to be done all over again.

Nothing can more certainly or more rapidly alter the state of the nutrition of the body than a fast. No other means at our disposal brings about a more rapid change in the chemistry of the body, especially of its fluids and secretions. Fasting relieves the pains of arthritis, for example, more effectively than drugs and does it without risk or harm.

The duration of the fast in arthritis will have to depend on individual circumstances and should never be undertaken except under the personal supervision of one who is thoroughly familiar with the techniques of fasting.

It is customary to advise the arthritic to exercise the affected joints to prevent these from becoming fixed. It is asserted that this stays the development of ankylosis or bony union. However much truth there may be in this claim, the forced activity tends to aggravate the inflammation and intensify the pain. I find it better to let the affected joint rest until fasting has enabled the body to remove the deposits and infiltrations from the joint and to clear up the inflammation. In this way the stiff joint spontaneously limbers up and may be used without pain.

The vast majority of patients with arthritis whom I have been called upon to care for have been in advanced stages of chronic disease. They have all had months to years of the usual forms of treatment, including the removal of several "foci of infection," and they have still suffered. Indeed, their history shows that they have grown progressively worse under such forms of treatment. They have been in pain. They were deformed.

They were more or less helpless. Why? I repeat: the primary cause of their suffering had been neglected.

Recovery from chronic arthritis is a slow evolution out of a state of ill health and into a state of biochemical dependability. It involves many factors—age, weight, extent of the disease, its duration, degrees of joint destruction, the amount of ankylosis, previous habits of living and eating, the amount of nerve energy in reserve, the character of complications that exist (such as heart disease), the occupation, disposition and environment of the patient. All of these factors determine the extent of recovery possible and the rapidity with which recovery can take place.

Chief among the requirements of recovery is a willingness and determination to carry out all instructions. Those who cheat and who balk at restrictions and rules are less likely to achieve the return of good health. An absolute minimum of sugar and starches should be included in the diet.

Self-control, self-denial, many restrictions, a dogged determination to get well, even if the restrictions are sometimes irksome and the progress discouraging, help in recovery.

progress discouraging, help in recovery.

23

Peptic Ulcer

When, on July 28, 1939, William J. Mayo, M.D., the last of the two brothers who established the famous Mayo clinic, died, the press carried the story that he died of a sub-acute perforating ulcer, an abdominal ailment he had specialized in treating. Said one dispatch: "Stricken shortly after he returned from a winter vacation in the southwest, Dr. Will underwent a stomach operation at the clinic last April and never fully recovered."

It was but a few years after Dr. Mayo's death when it was announced from this same clinic that operation for ulcer is not good treatment. While operations are still being performed for ulcers, they are not performed so frequently as formerly.

It is no unusual thing for a specialist to die of the disease in which he specializes. That they "take their own medicine" attests to their sincerity; that they cannot protect themselves reveals that the knowledge they possess is not dependable. A man may be a leading surgeon and not know the cause of the peptic ulcer, and endurated (hardened) pylorus, the fibroid tumor, the gallstone or kidney stone that he cuts out. This is a very unsatisfactory situation; without a knowledge of cause, the specialists is working in the dark.

The symptoms of "diseases of the stomach" are many—and often not nearly so clear-cut as the layman may imagine.

It is true there are a few more or less "fixed symptoms" of stomach ulcer—pain, tenderness at the pit of the stomach, vomiting and hemorrhage, but these may also be symptoms of cancer or they may be present in less serious diseases of the stomach. For these reasons diagnosis of ulcer from the symptoms alone is very difficult. X-ray and fluoroscopic examinations are made to confirm the examiner's suspicions, but it is only in exceptionally pronounced cases that this means can prove anything conclusively.

The fact is that the X-ray often indicates ulcer where no ulcer exists and often fails to reveal an ulcer where one does.

Falsely called an "executive's disease," peptic ulcer is said to kill 11,000 persons a year in this country, through hemorrhage and complications. Thirteen million Americans are said to have peptic ulcer. It may be open to serious doubt that there are that many executives in the nation. Abuses in eating, drinking, smoking, sex, the emotions, and in other facets of living are the most likely causes. Tilden says that "the sexually enervated are slow to reproduce tissue. Ulcers refuse to heal; infections slowly, but surely, take place; chronic diseases are uncontrollable." In the sexually abused there is laid the groundwork for the evolution of many diseases.

The prevailing concept is that peptic ulcer, that is, ulcer of the lower end of the esophagus, the stomach and of the upper end of the duodenum, is due to the action of the gastric juice (the hydrochloric acid and pepsin) of the stomach digesting and corroding the walls of these parts of the digestive tube. As the food is carried below the duodenum, bile and other juices render the content alkaline, so that there is no action of the pepsin and hydrochloric acid, hence no peptic ulcers below the duodenum.

This concept is far from being as certain as some believe. The membrane of the stomach is chemically non-corrosive. For untold ages the lining of these organs has been in contact with the digestive juices and this juice has been digesting the toughest protein foods that man has eaten and, normally, throughout all this time, the gastric juice has not digested the delicate lining of the stomach, esophagus and duodenum.

To say that suddenly the acid and pepsin of the stomach digests and corrodes the lining of these organs and let the matter rest there is to fail to understand the cause of peptic ulcer.

It is said that something happens to the internal chemistry of the body to cause the gastric juice to digest the stomach; it is believed, by some, that emotional stresses may be the cause of this chemistry change. Once the membrane collapses, so the theory runs, the stomach juice certainly acts on the tissues and extends the ulcer, often eating through the wall of the stomach or duodenum (perforation) with fatal results.

It is significant in this connection that this digestion that is assumed to be certain is an exceedingly slow process, often requiring years for its climax.

Yet this self-digestion does not occur in the healthy stomach, no matter how much acid may be secreted. Hydrochloric acid is a normal secretion of the glands of the stomach, a necessity in the digestion of protein foods. To believe that it is disease-building is not rational. An excess of acid secretion due to some evanescent cause may give rise to discomfort and distress, but there will be no digestion of the lining membrane of the stomach. There may be a flow of the contents of the stomach back into the gullet, resulting in the symptom commonly called "heart burn," but this will not result in any damage to the membrane.

Long-continued suffering with heart burn (most often seen in those who overeat on sugars and syrups and those who wrongly combine their foods, and who drink liquids with meals) may result in sufficient irritation of the lining of the esophagus and stomach to cause inflammation, but up to this point, at least, there will be no digestion of the walls of the gullet and stomach. The acids of decomposition, resulting from overeating and imprudent eating, are the acids that complicate gastric and duodenal ulcer.

Experimentally, fresh tissue from other parts of the body, when sutured to the gastric wall, is not digested and this suggests that the walls of the digestive tube are not digested by the gastric juice. But I think that an even stronger reason to doubt the role of the digestive juice in producing peptic ulcer is the fact that ulcers develop in many other part of the body—the nose, sinuses, mouth, tongue, throat, colon, bladder, womb, cervix, vagina, gall bladder and upon the surface of the body, as in varicose ulcer—without the digestive action of the gastric secretion.

There is in ulcers, in each of these other locations, a preliminary and persistent inflammation with hardening and a subsequent breakdown of tissue. The evaluation of ulcer of the esophagus, stomach and duodenum out of chronic irritation and inflammation and hardening seems to be as certain as its evolution out of these pre-ulcer states in other locations.

The history of cases of gastric and duodenal ulcer reveals that very early in life, the patient had developed gastro-intestinal irritation and inflammation. The mode of living and eating that resulted in the irritation continued, added to, intensified, and the recurring discomforts were palliated with drugs, until the patient passes through the already indicated stages of pathological evolution—irritation, inflammation, a gradual thickening of the mucous and sub-mucous tissues (hardening), and, then, ulceration.

The increasing hardening chokes arterial circulation, cutting off oxygen and the food supply, so that the tissues break down, giving rise to an open sore or ulcer.

Cancer may be the final ending in this evolution. It is one of the endings of a chain of symptoms starting with irritation, and passing through inflammation, thickening and swelling (hardening or induration), ulceration (ulcer formation), and fungation (cancer).

The same chain of causes and effects may precede both endings or cancer may evolve out of the ulcer. It should be understood that both of these diseases—ulcer and cancer—represent end-points in a process of pathological evolution that had simple beginnings and became more complex as it developed. This is the reason why the search for a specific cause for cancer has been so disappointing.

All of the cancer-producing (carcinogenic) agents so far discovered are causative in only a certain percentage of cases—in those in whom the ground has already been prepared for cancer development.

Ulcer, like cancer, is an ending in a chain of symptoms that begins far back of the evolution of the ulcer itself. Repeated stomach crises (gastritis) end in ulcer. The ulcer develops after scores of gastric crises that have occurred frequently in infancy, childhood, youth, and maturity. Ulcer is classed as an organic disease, which means that abnormal changes have taken place in the structure of the wall of the organ affected.

Organic changes follow in the wake of vascular (artery and vein) degeneration and hardening. Indurations (hardenings) wait upon circulatory changes, particularly asphyxiation of the tissues.

Ulceration may be said to be an active degeneration from cell apoplexy; cancer is passive degeneration from cell asphyxiation. The beginning of both these forms of disease is irritation. All chronic forms of inflammation begin as irritation and are followed by ulceration and, if the location favors stasis (stoppage of the blood flow), induration and cancer will follow.

The major links in this chain of pathological evolution are enervation, intoxication, irritation, inflammation, induration, ulceration and fungation. That last is cancer. Should cancer be the only unknown element in this pathological composite?

Concomitant with the gastric ulcer is a chronic state of excessive acidity of the stomach, a condition known as *gastric hyperacidity*. The common belief is that the excess stomach acid is a purely local condition.

It is not recognized that this hyperacidity is symptomatic of the systemic condition of the sufferer. This is the reason that treatment is only local; whereas, if it were recognized that the local state is but a phase of a constitutional state, a more rational and more successful plan of care could be instituted.

If the gastric irritation and inflammation continue, and they will if toxemia is not eliminated and its causes removed, the inflammation will extend to the gall duct and gall bladder and even into the liver itself. Or it may extend up the pancreatic duct into the pancreas. As the patient's mode of living is not corrected and the systemic condition back of the irritation and inflammation is increased and intensified, the disease spreads from membrane to membrane and new diseases develop.

Feeding the ulcer patient is a difficult problem. Not only is there a greatly impaired ability to digest food, but there is the irritation of the ulcerated surface that is occasioned by so many different foods.

What a life one leads when reduced to the necessity of conforming to the requirements of a capricious stomach! In peptic ulcer, due to the secretion of too much acid, it is customary to feed small, frequent meals of bland foods. These are intended to use up the acid and to reduce, as much as possible, the mechanical irritation of the ulcer.

But feeding the patient every three to four hours, sometimes oftener, and even at night, means that the patient is continually overeating. The very feeding program causes the excess secretion to be continued and helps to perpetuate the same condition it is intended to palliate. Using food as a palliative is certainly not a correct dietary procedure.

There are many different diets that are prescribed for ulcer patients and there are various plans of treatment. Each has its own advocates, but the results of each plan of care and feeding are far from satisfactory, for the reason that they ignore cause. Milk diets, cream diets, sippy diets, bland diets, frequent small meals, and similar feeding programs are all intended to palliate symptoms.

These diets cause less immediate irritation of the ulcerated surface, but they remove no cause, hence health is not restored. This is not a valid plan of feeding and it defeats its own purpose by adding to the systematic impairment that is back to the ulcer.

Drugs are also used to palliate symptoms—drugs to relieve pain, tranquilizers for depression, drugs to "coat the stomach," antacids to counteract the acidity. Other drugs employed in ulcer cases are intended only to provide short periods of relief from symptoms. They remove no cause, hence they restore no health. Even the latest method of freezing the glands of the stomach is but a palliative measure. It makes a digestive cripple out of the patient, but removes none of the causes of peptic ulcer.

Operations for peptic ulcer continue to be performed. And they are still very unsatisfactory. The wall of the stomach in gastric ulcer is pretty generally irritated and inflamed. In this broad field of inflammation the ulcer develops at the most inflamed point. This means that the part in which the greatest pathological change has occurred must ulcerate. Removing the ulcer does not remove the field of inflammation. Another point of the inflamed surface breaks down and another ulcer results.

This simply means that removal of an ulcer leaves the field open for the evolution of another ulcer and recurrence is the rule. Recurrence is due to the fact that the cause of the ulcer is untouched by the operation. Indeed, if the stomach is removed, and the cause untouched, trouble will evolve elsewhere out of the same causes. Surgery does not and cannot restore health. It is a means of palliating symptoms and rarely anything more. Anemia is a frequent aftermath of removal of large sections of the stomach.

Gastroenterostomy (formation of a connection or communication between the stomach and the small intestine, thus by-passing the pylorus) is a serious and crippling operation frequently performed where ulcer and thickening of the pylorus are suspected. It should be gratifying to know that it is not a necessary operation—that the thickened pylorus, like a thickened nasal membrane, can be thinned by the fast.

Fear and anxiety, coupled with the insistence of the surgeon that an operation is urgently needed, cause many patients to permit themselves to be rushed into an operation. The surgeon often paints vivid and frightening pictures of the dangers of delay. The equally startling post-operative picture is painted by one who has had the operation.

There is the operation, perhaps the subsequent operation for the relief of adhesions, the not infrequent gall bladder drainage or removal, a second or even a third operation on the stomach for recurrent ulcer, and the disillusionment that accompanies the return of symptoms. The disappointment and bitterness often shatter the patient's faith in medicine, but, alas! It comes too late.

The constitutional condition behind and preceding the incidence of peptic ulcer is by far the most vital factor involved in its evolution. The anemia frequently seen in ulcer patients is probably less due to the slight loss of blood through the ulcer than to the failure of blood making consequent upon the general nutritional impairment of the patient.

As the nutritive impairment precedes the formation of the ulcer often by several years producing in many instances the so-called "ulcer race" the original impairment is not to be blamed upon the ulcer. Everything in the condition of the patient, both those pathologies that precede the ulcer and those that are concomitant with it or successive to it, point to an existing constitutional impairment which forms the basis of the ulceration. This is one reason that purely local treatment of ulcers is so uniformly unsatisfactory.

Any sore (whether on the exterior of the body or on the inside skin—the membrane lining the digestive tract) will heal more rapidly and readily if unhampered. It must not continaully be irritated by handling, rubbing, wrinkling, contracting and expanding.

The irritation resulting from these mechanical activities, breaks down the healing tissues and causes bleeding. The sore will heal better if given rest. For this reason, the first step necessary to insure healing of a peptic ulcer is to ensure complete rest for the ulcerated organ. Nothing provides this local rest of the digestive organs more completely than the fast.

Irritation of the raw surface of the ulcer resulting from the gastric acidity will also prevent healing of the peptic ulcer. New tissue cannot form in the presence of such irritations. Since fasting causes a cessation of a secretion of gastric juice, which otherwise bathes the ulcerated surface, this source of irritation is removed by the fast. In most cases only about three days of fasting are required to suspend the secretion of gastric juice. The small amount of juice secreted thereafter will be very weakly acid.

Thus the fast speedily removes three sources of local irritation—the mechanical irritation brought on by particles of food in contact with the raw surface, mechanical irritation resulting from contraction and expansion of the walls of the stomach and wrinkling of its surfaces in receiving and handling foods, and chemical irritation caused by the acid gastric juice. With the removal of these sources of irritation, healing can proceed at a satisfactory rate.

But fasting has another and more profound effect in the restoration of health to the ulcer patient. "Since it is easy to demonstrate," wrote George Weger, M.D., "that the quckest way to overcome constitutional acidity and restore normal alkalinity is by an absolute fast while resting in bed, one can readily see that a complete fast serves not alone a dual purpose, but every purpose." He cautions against breaking the fast too soon, saying that this is a frequent cause of failure. *"The fast must be continued until all reactions indicate that systemic renovation has been completed."*

It is also important to know that the fast results in the thickened lining of the pylorus becoming thinned so that this passage again becomes normal, providing, of course, that this is done before scar tissue has formed. Fasting will not result in a removal of scar tissue. As there are stages of pathological evolution that cannot be remedied, it is the part of wisdom to remove all causes of disease and restore the tissues to a normal state before such irreversible stages are reached.

Pyloric inflammation will quickly improve and the patient will recover health if the habits of the patient, especially his eating habits, are corrected. While I have especially emphasized the necessity of correcting the habits of eating, it should be understood that all enervating habits should be discontinued.

Recovery from an ulcer involves far more than mere temporary healing of the ulcerated surface. Ulcers do heal and then recur, often doing so several times in the life of an ulcer patient. Ulcers are frequently surgically removed, only to recur. The fact that there have been numerous instances of recurrence after four and five operations for gastric ulcer is sure evidence that the operation does not restore health. It fails to remove cause and until this is done there can be no genuine recovery.

Restoration of good health can take place at every stage of the pathological evolution which I have pictured, from the irritation of the first cold to ulceration, inclusive, but when cachexia (the defining symptom of cancer) has evolved, the condition is irreversible.

"I know that my headaches are due to constipation," a sufferer with migrane told me one day. "I'm certain that if I could get rid of constipation, I would not suffer with headaches." She had suffered for years and had been the rounds of the disease-treaters. She had had about all the forms of treatment the various schools of healing could offer, but she had never received more than brief periods of evanescent relief.

I told her that she had the true picture reversed. If she would get rid of her headaches, she would be free of constipation. To this statement she replied: "You are crazy." I replied: "I know it, and so are you." She asked: "What do you mean?" Then I explained to her that headache is a symptom and constipation is a symptom and that symptoms do not cause each other, but that if she would get rid of the common cause of both symptoms, she would be free of both of them at the same time.

She accepted this as a logical approach to her troubles. No one else had ever suggested to her that it would be essential to remove the cause of her suffering in order to end the suffering. They had all depended on treatments to do what only removal of cause can do.

She had a relatively short fast to enable her encumbered body to unload its accumulated toxin and this was followed by a better way of living. She had no more headaches and her constipation ended at the same time.

Commonly referred to as "sick headache," and "bilious headache" migraine is defined as "periodic cephalalgia, (pain in the head), characterized by the absence of any local lesions which might cause headaches, and peculiar as regards the visual and oculoplegic symptoms and psychic symptoms which may accompany it." Standard medical works state that there is evidence to sustain the view that migraine is allergic in nature and I have even read the positive statement that it "can be shown to be hereditary in every instance."

Also called *megrim* and *hemicrania*, this *syndrome* is characterized by periodic headaches, often one-sided, and accompanied by nausea, vomiting, and various disturbances of the senses, particularly disturbances of the eyes and ears. There is also likely to be intolerance to light and noise, great prostration and an incapacity for mental concentration.

Few if any other so-called functional diseases are accompanied by so much suffering. Indeed, it is not an uncommon thing for these patients to become drug addicts in their search for relief from their symptoms.

Walter C. Alvarez, M.D., says that it is usual to put such patients in a hospital and give them every test known to science and that as always in cases of migraine, nothing is "found that could cause the migraine." This is in line with the usual statement in standard works that no cause for the disease is known.

Dr. Weger, on the other hand, makes a very profound observation in relation to the disease: "The toxemia theory can be more effectively demonstrated in its application to migraine than in diseases of less regular periodicity. Due to frequent recurrence and consequent opportunity for observation, every disease building factor can be checked and demonstrated in any given case so that the whole complex can be laid bare and uncovered to the understanding."

Women who have migraine (the disease is rare among men) are enervated and toxemic. They suffer with poor digestion, often with menstrual troubles, and congestion of the pelvis. It is not difficult to determine the relation of migraine to the menstrual function, pelvic congestion and other abnormal states of the reproductive organs. Poisoning coming from the digestive tract, added to the prior enervation and toxemia, quickly builds migraine in those who are predisposed to its evolution.

I recall a typical instance in which I told a woman with migraine that she could be made well—not *cured*—in a period of from four to six weeks. "I don't believe you," she stated. "Why should fasting help when nothing else has?"

I have heard similar statements many times in these cases. When she was relieved of the headaches, of course, she had no reason to disbelieve further. But in most of these cases, the sufferers have no ground in their past experience to give them hope that permanent relief can be achieved.

Certainly none of the mere palliative treatments in vogue have given any confidence.

Ergotamine and other "pain killing" drugs, as well as coffee freely used, to damage and fail to remove any causes.

It is rarely necessary for a sufferer with migraine to have more than a few headaches after she is started on a *Hygienic* program. Indeed, she is most likely to get rid of her aches while she is still fasting and they are not likely to recur when eating is resumed.

There are long-standing cases where the nervous systems have been badly impaired by nerve-depressing drugs. Here an extended period of strict self-discipline and a strong determination to stick to a healthful program is required if the individual is to recover fully.

Aside from such rather infrequent cases, most women can get well of their migraine by resort to a relatively short fast. But this must be followed by a genuine correction of living habits afterwards. Ten days to three weeks of fasting under experienced supervision, will suffice in most cases.

After-care also, in both the breaking of the fast and in the general return to good living habits, should be equally well supervised.

25

Hay Fever

The woman was an invalid. She had to be carried from bed to chair and from chair to bed. She was too weak to walk more than a few steps at a time. Among her several complaints was hay fever with which she had suffered each season for a number of years. It was 1918, and we were busy making the world safe for democracy.

Every Sunday she was taken by her husband to a Bible class. He would bring along a reclining chair for her to use during the class. It was at this Bible class that she met a *Hygienist* and was induced to try *Hygiene* as a means of recovering health. Weak as she was, she underwent not one but several short fasts.

Today as I write her story she has reached what many would consider old age, 73 years. She is in good health. She has been able to work through these decades. For more than forty years she has had no recurrence of hay fever. She has lived all of this time in southern climates where the air is filled with pollens almost all the year.

She has no allergies and eats any wholesome food that she desires. She is, however, but one among thousands who have recovered from hay fever by the unloading of toxins and correcting the mode of life.

In hay fever the Schneiderian membrane (a mucous membrane) of the nose becomes highly sensitive as a consequence of a state of chronic irritation (inflammation) for a lengthy period of time. Particles of dust, lint, and pollen, easily add to the irritation and cause it to "water" and become congested. The excited, irritated and inflamed state of the mucous membrane of the eyes, nose and throat seen in hay fever is but a state of what was formerly known as catarrh. To put this very simply: the sensitive condition of those membranes is due to the fact that they are sick—inflamed.

Today hay fever is said to be an allergy or to be caused by an allergy. Precise descriptions of allergy vary greatly. In general it is defined as "a condition of unusual or exaggerated specific susceptibility to a substance which is harmless in similar amounts for the majority of members of the same species."

Yet it seems to me to define allergy as an unusual sensitivity is to beg the question—and to explain nothing.

The baffled expert hides behind the brilliant obscurity of his definitions. Allergy is now said to be due to failure of one of the normal defense mechanisms of the body. If there is truth in this, it must not be permitted to blind us to the fact that the symptoms that are called allergic reactions represent the calling into play of another of the body's normal defense mechanisms. If one means of defense fails or is inadequate, there are other modes of defense at the command of the living organism which it may call upon. It is not left helpless because of the failure of one mechanism.

Whatever else we may think of allergy, we must recognize that it is not a self-caused state. Why is one man allergic and another not? Or, take the theory that allergy represents the failure of a defense mechanism, why does the defense mechanism of one fail while that of another does not? To answer this question, we return to our basic cause of disease—toxemia.

What is the cause of hay fever? It is a chronic inflammation of the nasal passages growing out of a pronounced toxemic condition that commonly has lasted for years. Toxemia is the basic cause of all inflammations of the lining membranes of the hollow organs of the body. So long as the toxemic state is maintained by enervating habits and so long as overeating is persisted in, there is no possibility of recovering from hay fever.

Anyone can test this statement for himself. Abstain from food for a time and watch the nasal discharge and other symptoms of hay fever clear up. There is simply no need for any one to go on, year after year, suffering with hay fever. Let the sufferer bear in mind that the pollens, the hair of animals, and other substances to which he is sensitive of allergic, are normal elements of his environment and he will realize that his sensitivity of them must be due to something within himself, rather than in those perfectly normal things that do not trouble other people. All of these elements are sources of allergic annoyance only to the sick. The healthy are not allergic.

The hay fever sufferer will cease to be troubled as soon as he is restored to health. He will not again be affected by them so long as he maintains a state of high level health. There are numerous means of palliating the symptoms of hay fever, but as none of these remove any causes, none restore the patient to health.

Each season he is forced to return to the means of palliation, to rush off somewhere to escape the source of his irritation. This is expensive, time-consuming and—futile.

The hay fever sufferer should take a real vacation: he should go to bed and abstain from food. This will be both less expensive and more effective than sea voyages or junkets to pollen-free mountains. Once the sufferer has been freed of his toxic load and the irritated state of the membranes of his eyes, nose and throat has been corrected, all symptoms of hay fever come to an end and they do not recur if he lives healthfully. Any return to enervating habits and to overeating will result in a recurrence of the hay fever.

The period of fasting required in hay fever is commonly longer than that required for the more simple ailments. The time will run, in the average case, from ten days to four or even five weeks. Overweight individuals will require a longer fast than those of average weight or less.

Allergy in hay fever, as well as in migraine headache, is not a cause but a symptom.

The answer in both instances lies in disintoxication by fasting, by cleansing, by proper modes of living.

26

High Blood Pressure

High blood pressure is said to be second to hardening of the arteries as a cause of heart disease in this country. By high blood pressure in this instance is meant that form of increased blood pressure that is called hypertension. Due to a narrowing of the arteries, pressure builds up behind the constricted vessels, thus adding to the work of the heart.

Blood pressure may be understood if we think of a water hose through which water is flowing. The water flows through the unobstructed hose with a certain degree of pressure. If a nozzle is put onto the hose, so that there is some obstruction to the flow of the water, there is an increase in water pressure. If the opening of the nozzle is reduced, the water pressure increases still more. The smaller the opening of the nozzle, the more water pressure is built up behind it.

The same thing occurs in the arteries, in what is known as *essential hypertension*. The aorta, the largest artery in the body, may be compared to a tree trunk. The main arteries branch off from this and other arteries branch off from these, like the branches of a tree. The branching continues, until some of the branches are so small that they may be regarded as the twigs of the arterial tree.

It is the narrowing or constriction of these arterioles that results in the building up of blood pressure. Far from being disease of old age, hypertension is frequently seen in the young, even, in rare instances, in babies.

It is estimated that today five million Americans suffer with some degree of hypertension. As the standards of normal blood pressure are not valid, the probability is that a far higher number of Americans than this figure indicates have high blood pressure of the hypertensive type. Perhaps in the vast majority of instances, the pressure is not high enough to constitute an annoyance or a hazard, but its tendency is to increase with time. In no case should its causes be neglected.

It is essential that we recognize the fact that high blood pressure is an ending in a chain of causes and effects that extend back in the life of the patient for years—tensions in business and personal affairs over-taxing the nervous system.

Excessive venery is one of the most prominent causes, but lasciviousness when it is in control of the mind is equally as pernicious. Excessive eating, coffee, tea, tobacco, alcohol, and a lack of poise are among the most common causes. Salt eating undoubtedly contributes to its production, but to blame high blood pressure on this alone is to ignore all the many other influences in the life of the patient.

In traditional Alice in Wonderland fashion of starting with a result as a cause, hypertension is said to cause heart disease, and the hypertension is blamed upon the nerves.

The fact that substances liberated by the kidneys, by the adrenal glands, perhaps substances liberated by the thyroid and pituitary glands, can also cause high blood pressure, tends to reveal that the condition may be more than simple nerve irritation—that it is a symptom of a general or systemic state. This being true, the remedy is not some temporary forced reduction of pressure, but a thorough removal of the causes of systemic impairment.

Treatment is commonly directed to depressing the nervous system. The surgical procedures of removing the thyroid gland and portions of the sympathetic nervous system are both based on the assumption that the organs of the body are causes of disease. The fact that high blood pressure never develops spontaneously in animals is given as the reason for the thought that the nervous system is involved in the cause of hypertension in man.

Drugs given to depress the nervous system, to relax the arterial system, and to depress the heart are the most common means of reducing blood pressure in cases of hypertension. It hardly needs to be pointed out that such treatment removes no cause and provides reduction to the pressure only so long as the drugs are being taken.

Indeed, in most cases, the blood pressure tends to rise in spite of the depressing effects of the drugs, after they have been taken over a brief period. The drugs all result in more or less annoying and often serious side effects, so that there is a constant search for new, and it is hope, less injurious drugs. Certainly the treatments in vogue are not satisfactory, neither to the patients nor to their physicians.

Multiple causation makes specific treatment a tragedy. The remedy must be as many-sided as the cause. It will not do, for example, to have the patient discontinue the eating of salt and permit him to continue to indulge in tobacco. Every element of cause must be removed to achieve certain and lasting results. We should also recognize the fact that in high blood pressure we deal with a symptom of a general systematic state that has been years in the making and is the result of many correlated antecedents.

The whole of the systemic abnormality must be remedied if we are to be successful in our efforts to provide permanent reduction of blood pressure. Treatment directed at the symptom cannot do more than provide a brief palliation of the symptom.

The speed with which fasting results in a marked reduction of blood pressure indicates the importance of rest in reducing systemic tension and excitement. The reduction may be so great in a very few days as to astonish the patient. As the toxic load is reduced, the nervous system becomes less irritated, the functions of the kidneys, adrenal, thyroid and pituitary glands are restored to normal, so that blood pressure falls to new levels, even to normal or slightly below, and tends to remain down after eating is resumed. Indeed, it will remain at or about the normal level so long as the patient continues to live in a manner to avoid the redevelopment of toxemia.

All of this is to say that the reduction of blood pressure secured by means of the fast is a genuine reduction and not a forced state. The organism is not crippled in the process as it is when a gland or portions of the sympathetic system are removed. If we cut out causes instead of cutting out organs, we secure a genuine and lasting elimination of effects.

As in all things, the causes that have produced the condition in the first place, will reproduce it if they are not permanently removed. Fasting is not a substitute for achieving—and holding to a correct way of life.

27

The Fast and the Heart

It was formerly widely held by physicians that if one were to go without food for six days the heart would collapse and death would result. The myth that fasting causes the heart to collapse persisted in scientific circles, in spite of the great amount of evidence to the contrary, until after the famous Cork hunger strike in 1920.

Protesting their arrest following the Easter Rebellion of Irish patriots, Terence Mac Swiney, Lord Mayor of Cork, Ireland, and his co-fasters went without food for periods ranging from over seventy days to ninety-four days. They demonstrated by their long fasts the fallacy of the "heart collapse" from the lack-of-food theory.

Today we are foced to recognize the fact that instead of fasting weakening the heart, it results in strengthening this wonderful organ.

Stunt or exhibition fasters had also shown that man may safely abstain from food for extended periods and their sensational proofs had received sufficient publicity, even scientific study, to have dispelled the fallacy. Indeed, fasts by early *Hygienists* demonstrated the fallacy of this idea of the early collapse of the heart, years before it was abandoned in the world of science.

On this subject, Hereward Carrington, Ph.D., author of *Vitality, Fasting* and Nutrition says: "That the heart is invariably strengthened and invigorated by fasting is true beyond a doubt. I take the stand that fasting is the greatest of all strengtheners of weak hearts—being, in fact, its only rational physiological care." He attributed this improvement to the following three factors:

1. The added rest for fast provides for the heart.
2. The resulting improvement of the blood-stream.
3. The absence of the "stimulants" that patients in general and heart patients in particular are accustomed to take.

If we consider angina pectoris, a disease of the heart that grows out of constant stimulation with tobacco, coffee, tea, wrong food combinations and excesses of carbohydrates, and observe the effects of the fast in these patients, we are amazed at the speed with which the heart recovers from its difficulties.

Individuals who are inclined to overeat greatly, who have not learned their limitations regarding quantity and who tend to overdo everything they undertake are likely to develop angina pectoris. Their mode of living places a heavy and constant strain upon the heart. Rest is its most urgent need.

It is said authoritatively that during the past twenty years more than fifty drugs and surgical treatments have been advocated for the relief of angina pectoris. At the same time angina has been called a "self-limited disease," and some authorities have held the position that their advice tried during recovery might get the credit.

How do we know that fasting is of genuine value in a case of angina? We do not claim that fasting *cures* angina. We state only that it takes a load off the heart so that it may restore it own normal condition in a more certain and speedy manner.

"The ticker has certainly improved and slowed down; I can't hear it any more," this was a blind Canadian discussing his condition with me after a few days of fasting, followed by a few days of eating. Before beginning the fast he told me that for some time he had been able to hear the beat of his heart and that it was especially bothersome at night when he laid his head on the pillow.

There was also rapid heart action, which troubled him considerably. Nothing brings about a quieting down of a rapid heart and an excited system generally like rest with fasting. This takes a heavy load off the heart and results in a speedy reduction of blood pressure.

With a reduction of tension and a reduction of the number of repetitions of the heart's pulsations, this remarkable organ secures a real rest, something that nothing else can provide. With less work to do, the heart repairs itself.

The fast, as has been repeatedly emphasized in the preceding pages, is a period of physiological rest. It does not do anything, it is merely a cessation of doing. The rest provides opportunity for the body to do for itself, under conditions of rest, what it cannot do under conditions of full-speed ahead.

It can perform under abstinence what it cannot manage in a state of surfeit. So regular and uniform is the improvement of the heart in the fast that it cannot be doubted that Carrington's statements are true. There are, of course, heart conditions that are beyond any possibility of improvement and these will not be helped by the fast.

In the hundreds of cases of heart disease that I have watched through fasts of various lengths, all but a few have developed stronger and better hearts. Many of them, even so-called *incurable* ones, have become entirely normal. Rapid hearts have slowed down, abnormally slow hearts have speeded up, weak hearts have greatly improved in vigor, hearts that were irregular have become regular in time and frequency, hearts that were missing pulsations (even as often as one pulsation out of four) have resumed regular pulsation, and many other improvements in heart function have been observed. (It should not be necessary to say that fasting does not enable the heart to grow a new valve where one had been destroyed.)

Since fasting relieves the heart of a great burden, improvement should not be surprising. The heart is nourished from the body's nutritive reserves just as certainly, and often more adequately, than from raw materials arriving daily from the digestive tract. What more natural than that, given the rest that fasting provides, it should be able to repair itself and renew its functional vigor?

The rest provided for the heart is accounted for in two primary ways:

1. *There is a marked lessening of the number of pulsations of the heart.* A heart that is pulsating eighty times a minute will fall to sixty or even fewer beats a minute. If the heart is pulsating at a more rapid rate than eighty a minute, the fall in the pulse rate is even more dramatic.

If we use the first figure of eighty pulsations a minute to work from and take the figure of sixty beats a minute to represent the level to which the pulsations fall, we have a saving of twenty pulsations a minute or twelve hundred pulsations an hour or 28,800 pulsations in twenty-four hours. This represents a great reduction in the amount of work the heart does.

Of course there are the usual fluctuations of the heart rate due to exertion and emotion.

2. *Another restful factor is the fall of blood pressure*. If the pressure is 160 mm. it will speedily fall to 140, 130, even 115, where it will remain for the rest of the period of fasting. I saw one case of a woman who had a systolic pressure of 295 mm. in which the pressure was reduced in less than two weeks to 115 mm. This means that the heart is working against lessened resistance. It beats with less force. Less forceful pulsations coupled with reduced number of pulsations provide a rest for the tired and impaired heart. Under such conditions it repairs and strengthens itself, and in a good number of cases that have been declared to be *incurable*, the heart has been fully restored.

I call the foregoing sources of heart rest, *primary*. There are other sources of rest for the heart that may be called *secondary*. First among these is the reduction of weight. This is most marked in fat individuals whose size is such that the heart has to labor to keep the blood circulating through so much bulk. While the pressure often falls in these cases more rapidly than the flesh is lost, the loss of pounds relieves the long-suffering heart of a burden. Every pound that is lost relieves the heart of work it has been forced to do.

Another factor to consider is that, in decompensation, the fall in the rate of pulsation is not as immediate and rapid as in ordinary fasting cases.

Decompensation is the inability of the heart to maintain adequate circulation. It is characterized by difficult breathing (dyspnea) blueness of the lips and fingers (cyanosis) rapid, but feeble heart actions, venous engorgement, a decreased urinary output, with, in severe cases, an accumulation of fluid in the tissues—edema, dropsy, anasarca.

Although already greatly weakened, the increased work of the heart occasioned by the accumulating fluid, adds to its difficulties. The heavier burden on the heart becomes intolerable and it slowly weakens under the load. As the heart weakens the dropsy increases and as this increases, the work of the heart is increased. A vicious cycle is established from which it is difficult to escape.

Another source of edema is the taking of common table salt (sodium chloride). This salt is non-usable and poisonous. It is excreted with difficulty, hence it tends to accumulate in the body of the salt-eater. It is stored in the surface tissues just under the skin and in cavities, along with water that is needed to dilute it, thus forming brine. This salt-occasioned edema, often sufficiently marked in supposedly healthy individuals to be easily detected (in others existing as a hidden edema) places an added burden upon the heart and kidneys.

The body of the fasting patient is able to bring the salt and water back into the circulation, from where it is excreted. There is commonly an enormous urinary excretion of sodium chloride, in such cases, up to 78 grams of salt a day having been observed to be excreted during a fast. It has been shown by careful biochemical observations that fasting results in an absolute increase in the amount of sodium chloride excreted, even in cases in which the total urinary output is small.

As the sodium chloride content of the blood remains normal during the fast, the indication is that the salt excreted is from the edema and effusion flud accumulation.

The first step in the excretion of the salt-water accumulation is the return of the water and salt to the blood stream. Fasting favors the absorption of the fluid from the tissues and its subsequent excretion. When the fast is instituted and all intake of salt is entirely discontinued, the body is enabled to rapidly withdraw the water and sodium chloride from the edematous tissues. The hidden edema and dropsy disappear at a rapid rate.

The principle of lightening the work of the circulatory system and particularly that of the heart by decreasing the food intake and by eliminating salt from the diet is carried to its ultimate stage when the heart patient fasts. Often it is even found necessary to reduce greatly the amount of water taken. Especially in cases of marked edema (dropsy) is it important to reduce the water intake in order to facilitate the excretion of the fluid from the tissues.

In decompensation of the heart, there is commonly renal (kidney) stasis—stoppage of the blood flow—which impairs the function of the kidneys. The fast seems to result in an instantaneous improvement in the function of the kidneys, so that there is an immediate increase of elimination. There are different views about water intake in this condition, some fasting advocates favoring taking water freely, on the theory that the kidneys can function better if plenty of water is taken; others holding that the intake of liberal quantities of water slows down the excretion of the edematous accumulation. I favor limiting water intake.

With the increased excretion, through the kidneys, of water and sodium chloride, so that the edema is reduced or obliterated, the heart is greatly relieved. It has also been suggested that fasting may favorably affect certain vaso-motor centers, (the nerve centers that control circulation), thus causing improvement in the condition of the heart and arteries.

Certainly it would be folly to say that the excretion of water and sodium chloride in dropsical conditions is alone responsible for the wide relief of symptoms that occur. The concomitant general improvement of the heart and circulatory condition must be taken into full consideration, but there is reason to think that the increased urinary outpout and the absorption of water and salt from the tissues is due, in great measure, to the improvement of the general circulatory action, the improvement tending to persist after eating is resumed.

An Italian physician, Giorgio Dagnini, M.D., studied the results of fasting in sixteen cases of cardiac decompensation and presented a detailed account of his observations in the *Institute of General Medicine and Therapeutics* of the University of Modena, Italy. I am indebted to an American physician, who is interested in fasting, for an English translation of the account.

Dagnini says of these sixteen cases, many of whom had previously proved "refractory of therapy with cardiac drugs," that all of them suffered with severe cardiac decompensation. In addition to the fast, the patients were all given bed rest and all the water desired but no drugs. Twelve of these patients suffered with edema of the serous cavities; four had no edema.

Of the twelve edematous patients the clinical diagnoses were myocardial sclerosis (hardening of the heart muscle) in six cases; mitral stenosis (narrowing or stricture of the mitral valve of the heart) in two cases; mitral and aortic stenosis (stenosis of both the mitral and aortic valves) in one case; mitral insufficiency (failure of the mitral valve to close) in one case; malignant hypertension and cardiac asthma in one case; hypertension and cardiovascular disease, fibrillation and myocardial sclerosis in one case.

Both sexes were involved and their ages ranged from 24 years to 75 years. The fasts ranged from five days (the shortest) to seven days (the longest). Of the non-edematous group, three had mitral stenosis, one had hypertension with myocardial sclerosis. There was but one man in this group. The youngest of the group was thirty-eight years, the oldest, sixty-four years. These patients all fasted seven days.

All the fasts in these heart cased were short, but Dagnini says: "It was consistently observed that cardiac patients treated with fasting show increased urinary output and a rapid resorption of edema fluid and peritoneal and pleural effusions." In the non-edematous group sodium chloride excretion was about "normal." This may indicate that the edema in the other cases was as much the result of salt-eating as of heart weakness.

From among his twelve edematous patients, I would like to cite one case only, to picture the developments as they occur when a cardiac patient is fasted.

The patient was a twenty-four-year-old man who had a clinical diagnosis of mitral stenosis. He was in a grave condition, with failure largely on the right side of his heart. The heart was much enlarged in all diameters. The liver was enlarged to the iliac crest (the crest of the hip bone). There was slight effusion into the pleura, edema of the lower extremities and slight difficulty in breathing. Previous to admission to the institution this patient had been treated with the usual heart medicines.

At the institution he was given a fast of seven days. By the third day there was distinct improvement in his condition. The liver shrank at the surprising rate of two-finger-breadths a day. The edema fluid was rapidly absorbed through the fast. By the end of the seventh day the liver was but three fingerbreadths below the ribs and the generalized edema had disappeared.

There was much improvement of the pleural effusion. The urinary output in this case was significant. Being but 250 cc at the outset, it increased rapidly until by the fifth day it reached 3700 cc and remained at about 2000 cc thereafter. The diuresis in this case accounted for the removal of the edema.

Dagnini's observation that fasting has been employed beneficially in many types of cardiac decompensation and that this has suggested that its benefits are drawn, not from a single one of its effects, but from multiple effects, is worthy of careful consideration.

He suggests that "possibly many diverse effects are summed and potentiated with a resulting restoration of normal or near-normal cardiovascular function." Unfortunately his fasts were of short duration, never long enough for complete results, and he fails to tell us how they were followed up—how the patients were fed after the fast, what activities they were permitted, what subsequent developments resulted. But his observations, limited as these cases were, certainly, so far as the length of the fasts were concerned, are enough to reveal the beneficial effects of the fast in a wide, variety of severe heart abnormalities.

The intelligent individual will employ the fast long before his heart condition reaches the stage represented in the cases described by Dagnini. In spite of the benefits described, there is no doubt that these were terminal cases and no genuine recovery could have been expected in any of them.

The fast should be employed at a time when there is still possibility of genuine recovery.

I should not have to add, again, that it should be undertaken under competent and experienced direction and supervision, but the warning is important in these cases. No sufferer from heart disease—or the possible incipient stages of heart disease—should ever attempt to fast on his own.

Colitis is inflammation of the colon.

To understand what the colon is let us examine a brief physiological description. Anatomically, the human colon or large bowel, which is often likened to a sewer, is divided into three distinct sections: the ascending, transverse and descending colon. It begins with a blind pouch, the cecum, where the small intestine ends. The vermiform appendix is attached to the cecum. Immediately above the appendix, the cecum receives the small intestine, almost at right angles.

The upper end of the cecum merges into the first part of the ascending portion of the colon. This passes upward on the right side to a point near the liver, where an angle is formed (the hepatic flexure) and the second portion, the transverse colon, begins.

The transverse colon passes in a slight curve across the abdomen immediately under the stomach and, at the left side forms another angle (the splenic flexure). Below the spleen, the colon becomes the descending colon, which merges into the sigmoid flexure, and curves irregularly downward in an S shape. Between the end of the small intestine (the ileum) and the cecum, there is a valve formed by a sphincter muscle and known as the ileo-cecal valve. At the end of the rectum, another such valve (the rectal sphincter) closes the rectum.

The colon functions by carrying the residues of digestion upward from the cecum, across the transverse colon, and downward through the sigmoid to the rectum and to the outside world. Digestion is completed in the small intestine and it is there that the digested portions of the food are absorbed. Some water may be absorbed from the colon, but the small intestine is specially adapted for the absorption of food. There seems to be no absorption of toxins from the colon.

The colon, like all the rest of the alimentary tract, is lined with a skin or membrane that is called *mucous membrane*. Irritation, or inflammation of the colon is known as colitis or colonitis. Supposed by some authorities to be perhaps the most common disease of cilivized man, colitis is asserted to be very rare among uncivilized peoples. Constipation is perhaps the most annoying symptom of colitis, although it is likely to be alternated with diarrhea. If the colitis is acute (diarrhea) there may be mucus in the loose, watery stools. All the forms of colitis discussed in this chapter come under the general technical classification of "mucous colitis."

A state of spasm of the colon is common in cases of colitis, especially if the condition is marked. Frequently, also there is a sagging of the transverse colon—*enteroptosis*. The colon may sag in the absence of colitis and colitis may exist without sagging, but spastic colitis is almost certain to accompany both conditions.

It is a mistake,however, to think of the spastic constipation as the cause of the mucous colitis. This view is no more rational than to think of the colitis as the cause of the spastic constipation.

In chronic colitis the more marked inflammation may be located at different parts of the colon, the acute exacerbations of which will be named after the location of the more severe inflammation, as sigmoiditis, proctitis, etc.

For long periods the condition may be obscure, the individual merely being conscious of abdominal distress, which he may attribute to constipation or to gas. When mucus appears in the stools, the condition is already well advanced. As the colitis becomes more marked the mucus may appear in the stools in masses of jelly-like consistency, in suspicious looking ropy shreds like casts of the bowels, or the feces may be coated with mucus and this may be streaked with blood. There is now no mistake that colitis is present.

I do not intend here to attempt to cover all the variations from the common picture of colitis. These may occur, often, but for all practical purposes, they are of little significance. As the colon is divided into a few sections, it becomes possible to have such special forms of colitis as proctitis, sigmoiditis and others, but the so-called disease is the same in each case.

Let us look at the two "diseases" just named. There is no actual dividing line between the sigmoid and the rectum. If we imagine a hair line dividing the two continuous sections of the colon, we may recognize the folly of naming inflammation on one side of this line sigmoiditis, and, if it extends only an eighth of an inch over the line into the lining membrane of the rectum, calling this proctitis. It is like naming pimples on the left cheek one disease and pimples on the right cheek something else.

We make the same confusing classifications of inflammation according to locations throughout all parts of the body. Inflammation of the lining membrane of the nose is rhinitis, inflammation of the lining membrane of the nasal sinuses is sinusitis, inflammation of the bronchial tube is bronchitis; but these are only different names for precisely the same condition in the different locations. Gastritis is the same condition in the lining membrane of the stomach. To call all of these local inflammations different diseases is only to add to growing confusion.

Often great skill is needed to diagnose correctly the form of colitis with which the patient suffers, and to detect just where the inflammation is located. Skill in diagnosis may not indicate familiarity with cause. The greatest diagnostic technique is often harnessed to the most ineffective means of mere palliation.

We are here more interested in what is causing the patients trouble than in what particular section of the colon may be irritated or spastic. Symptoms of colitis are alike in kind, differing only in location and degree. One significant fact that has received much notice is that every case that presents the marks of chronicity has a *colon* complex; this is to say a negative or depressive *psychosis*.

People who are ill or who suffer are rarely cheerful and happy. Anxiety, apprehension and consequent depression form the rule in sickness of every nature. It is rarely possible for one to remain mentally or emotionally indifferent to physical discomfort. A certain measure of self-pity creeps into the consciousness of the most sanguine and stoical. When we consider the nature of colitis, it is not surprising that the sufferer becomes depressed and anxious. Many so-called *neurotics* and *psychotics* are such only because of long standing colitis.

In at least ninety-five percent of cases of chronic colitis, constipation is an outstanding feature. It frequently continues over a period of years, during which time the sufferer tries laxatives, purgatives, teas, oils, enemas, colonic irrigations, and other means of securing "relief" from his constipation, never once realizing that the constipation is only a symptom. Although these measures often afford some temporary relief, they serve, in the end, to aggravate greatly the condition.

All colitis sufferers complain of indigestion, both gastric and intestinal, and of rumbling of gas in the intestines, with more or less pain, sometimes of a colicy nature. They have a sense of fullness and uneasiness. Commonly there is a dull and constant or sharp and intermittent headache. Many of these patients complain of a feeling of stiffness and tension, even pain, in the muscles of the neck, often with pain just below the juncture of the neck and the head.

Frequently they describe their symptoms as a "drawing sensation." Most of these cases appear anemic and dysemic. They are thin and undernourished, as a rule, although colitis is by no means confined to the poorly nourished. The tongue is commonly coated, the taste unpleasant, and the breath offensive.

There may be a feeling of extreme exhaustion, with a lack of enterprise and ambition. Nausea may develop immediately upon the expulsion from the colon of a large accumulation of mucus. Invariably this is followed by a feeling of great relief.

In colitis the facial expression is one of dejection and misery, frequently combined with anxiety, although many try bravely to repress their feelings, while others appear to be in a constant state of unconcealed apathy. The patient may become very nervous, irritable, excitable, even border on melancholia and hysteria.

Not only a trial to themselves, they become a trial to everyone about them. In severe and long standing cases, the patient's whole thinking centers on his physical state. Few conditions can compete with colitis in engineering obsessions.

Many colitis sufferers become habituated to the taking of drugs. They try everything that is advertised as a remedy. They exhaust the list of laxatives, cathartics, tonics and digestants. They go from one physician to another, studying their symptoms and confusing their feelings. Enemas, cascades, irrigations, different methods of dieting, and psychiatrists are all tried in vain. Some study anatomy, physiology and foods and acquire an extensive technical vocabulary, often quite meaningless.

It has been suggested more than once that the milder types of insanity often have their origin in colonic irritation. At least mental diseases requiring restraint have evolved in colitiis sufferers. Such cases at least make it clear that the mental *reactions* to colitis are real and not mere fancies. One man of great prominence gives as his opinion that a chronically diseased colon forms the basis of more mental and physical troubles than any other single functional abnormality.

Most important in caring for the sufferer with colitis is to ignore symptoms and the acute exacerbations, and to recognize and remove the cause of the suffering. We are fully convinced that the development of colitis is concomitant with the retention of toxic waste and its accumulation in the blood and lymph. Whatever will free the body of its accumulated toxic load will prove adequate care for the colitis sufferer.

The mind of the patient and the mind of the one who cares for him must both be freed from the tyranny of local symptoms. The discomforts must be persistently minimized for the reason that the mucus, the gas, the rumbling, the spasticity, the constipation, and the nervous irritability, are neither singly nor collectively the cause of the trouble.

Recovery cannot be expected without complete and prolonged rest, away from friends and relatives and away from the enervating environmental factors. Physical rest means going to bed and remaining there. It means ceasing physical activities and relaxing. Mental rest requires poise. It means the elimination of worry, fear, anxiety, and depressing emotions. Sensory rest requires quiet and freedom from sensory excitement. Physiological rest can be obtained only by going without all food. Fasting soon results in a relaxation of the spastic bowel and stomach.

Instead of bulk-free diets, a fast is indicated. Fasting speeds up that part of metabolism that eliminates waste and rejuvenates fatigued nerve and cell structure. It permits the body to establish a normal blood chemistry in its own inimitable manner. No man understands how to establish a normal blood chemistry. No one can either duplicate or imitate the ways of the body in re-establishing its normal blood chemistry.

The continual irritation of the bowels by drugging can only add to the suffering of the patient, as this makes the condition worse. Medicated enemas are highly irritating. Enemas containing soapsuds, molasses and other such substances are also to be condemned.

It is important to know that colitis is but a part of a general irritation and inflammation of the mucous surfaces of the body (it would have been called but a few years ago, a general catarrh) and that whatever frees the patient of his colitis will, at the same time, free him of his other *itises* in other regions—in the nose and throat, in the womb or in the bladder, to name a few local mucous membrane inflammations.

The common condition called diarrhea is simply a colitis of short duration. Not serious in the average case, and lasting but a day or two (to a few days) it is the rule of many to neglect the state of the colon and resort to means of suppressing the diarrhea. Often the condition is nothing more than a temporary irritation of the bowels by unsuitable or fermenting food. This is especially true when it develops in children. But repeated crises of this kind tend to evolve chronic colitis.

As long ago as 1918, Richard C. Cabot, M.D., of Harvard University Medical School and the Massachusetts General Hospital, wrote in his book for social workers, *A Layman's Handbook of Medicine:* "Simple diarrhea or acute colitis of adults gets well as a rule in a week or ten days. The important remedies are rest and warmth and starvation." He indicates that this same care is best for infants and children, although he thought that a purge at the outset of the diarrhea should help. The impotant thing for us to note, however, is the recognition of the value of the fast in diarrhea. I think it should be added that a week to ten days constitutes more time than is required for most cases of diarrhea to come to an end if fasting is instituted at the first sign of diarrhea. Often two or three days are enough.

Amoebic dysentery is a form of colitis that is said to be caused by an amoeba. It is quite common in many parts of the world and I have had opportunity to handle a number of cases coming to me from Mexico and South America. I do not think that the dysentery is caused by the amoeba, but I am convinced that the amoeba and the medication aimed at this microbe tend to perpetuate a disease that, initially is but a simple inflammation of the bowel. The disease would "run its course" in a week to ten days in almost all cases, if not complicated by feeding and drugging.

When the true cause of the disease is understood and removed a speedy return to health follows, but if these cases are treated in the usual manner, the disease may last for years and end in death. Drugs to kill the amoeba, medicated enemas to kill parasites—these build ulcerative colitis and proctitis. The fact is that the war that is supposed to be made on the amoeba too often kills the patient before the *disease is controlled*. Some day amoebicides, parasiticides and germicides will be given up as they tend to kill the patient.

Instead of making war on the amoeba, the fast provides an opportunity for the body to cast off its nutritive redundancy and its toxic load and the diarrhea comes to an end. Whatever part the amoeba plays in the causation of the disease, it cannot be specific nor can it be primary, as this microbe ceases to annoy when the fast has progressed for a few days.

Two lovely young girls of the same family, citizens of this country, but living with their parents in Mexico City, where the father was stationed, developed a sickness diagnosed as amoebic dysentery, a disease very common in Mexico.

They had been treated in the regular manner: Drugs to kill the amoeba and plenty of "good nourishing food." In spite of the drugs, perhaps because of them, the dysentery persisted; in spite of the nourishing food, they continued to lose both weight and strength. Their parents began to despair of their lives. They knew of deaths in the disease in Mexico and began to fear that they were going to lose both of their daughters.

Then a New Yorker visited the family. He told them of *Hygiene* and urged them to give it a chance to restore the health of the two girls. The mother brought them to this country, where they were given a fast of only one week each.

The diarrhea ceased, they became more alert and developed a demand for food. The sisters were fed on a diet of fresh fruits, non-starchy vegetables and minimum quantities of proteins and carbohydrates. Their recovery was rapid and they put on weight on a diet that would not ordinarily sustain weight. Now after the passage of more than fifteen years, these two young ladies are still enjoying excellent health.

Ulcerative colitis is but a further evolution of mucous colitis. The chronic inflammation has resulted in hardening and ulceration of the membrane of the colon. Severe ulcerative cases may evolve out of acute colitis, but this is not the rule. Those who carry out the instructions given for mucous colitis will not evolve ulcerative colitis.

In a syndicated newspaper article published Oct. 24, 1962, Walter C. Alvarez, M.D., whom I have already quoted in this work, declared that chronic ulcerative colitis is "unfortunately . . . a disease which we physicians do not understand well. We don't know for sure what causes it." He explains that no germ or virus has been found that can be blamed as causing the often severe diarrhea and says that some cases seem certain to start with a nervous cause, such as an unhappy marriage. He adds that some physicians are sure that the disease begins and is kept going by "an allergic sensitiveness to some food or foods." Then he says: "However it starts, it often ends with a bad ulceration of the inner lining of the large bowel."

The patient develops fever, there is diarrhea with blood and pus in the feces, and, eventually, the colon shrinks and becomes deformed and shortened. In ulcerative colitis constipation frequently alternates with diarrhea. This condition may evolve after years of suffering with chronic colitis or it may evolve immediately after a severe acute inflammation of the colon.

In either case, it is correct to say that when colitis has passed through the successive stages of irritation, inflammation, ulceration and induration, it is ready for the evolution of cancer, which needs but the addition of a continuous bath of decomposition from excess and unsuitable food. It is essential to understand that all chronic forms of inflammation begin with irritation, followed by inflammation and ulceration. If the location favors stasis—stoppage of the blood flow—induration and cancer follow. In its origin irritation is absolutely innocent of all taint of malignancy, hence there is no reason why it cannot be remedied.

When ulcerative colitis is established cancer is not far away. Indeed, the objective symptoms of cancer and ulcer are far from pathognomic—that is, undeniably proving the presence of either. But there seems to be no reason to doubt that eating to the point of keeping the colon and rectum saturated with putrefaction is the one and only way to complete the evolution of cancer of the bowel. The beginning of the trouble is simply inflammation, which is absolutely innocent of all taint of malignancy until the diseased membrane of the colon or rectum has been mascerated, so to speak, in a continuous bath of decomposition.

The care of chronic inflammation of the colon and rectum should be successful at any stage before the beginning of malignancy. After the malignant stage is reached, hope flies out the window. This is to say, when colon disease has evolved through irritation, inflammation, ulceration, and induration to cancer, any remaining possibility of recovery is wrecked by methods of diagnosis and treatment that set up psychosis or mental depression as deadly as cancer itself.

Operation for cancer of the rectum or colon, making an artificial anus above the cancer, a questionable palliation, creates a blind pouch out of the cancerous portion of the colon or rectum, thus producing a miniature gehenna within the patient's body.

Alvarez says: "In a few cases, if no medical treatment helps, as the last resort the colon can be removed surgically." The drug treatment he describes is purely symptomatic: barbiturates to enable the patient to sleep, copavin or codeine to "quiet" the bowels and "give rest," extra fluids, and "some iron" for his anemia. He recommends antibiotics and cortisone-like drugs for other symptoms. One gets the idea that "treat the symptoms as they arise" is still *good medicine*.

Reverting to the article by Alvarez, he also says: ". . . The patient should be kept in bed a while, on a liberal diet, and one tasty enough so that he will eat it, and not leave it on his plate. He must have enough food and vitamins so that he can keep up his nourishment."

This is a slightly different way of expressing it, but what he says is only a restatement of the old advice that the patient must "eat plenty of nourishing food to keep up his strength." Eating prevents the bowel from healing and keeps alive the disease process. If the fast were instituted at the outset of the diarrhea, the formation of the ulceration could perhaps be avoided.

The remainder of the advice as to treatment which is given by Alvarez may prove enlightening. He says: "He will probably need barbiturates so that he can sleep at night, and he should have copavin, or codeine, to quiet his bowels and give him rest. He may need extra fluids, and he may need some iron for his anemia. One authority on this disease, Dr. J. A. Bargen of the Scott & White Clinic of Temple, Texas, gives an antibiotic, Azulfidine, which helps in some cases. Dr. Kirsner, of the University of Chicago, Dr. Ingelfinger, of Boston, and other authorities get results in some cases by giving cortisone-like drugs for a while. In a few cases, if no medical treatment helps, as a last resort the colon can be removed surgically."

Apparently from this, the authorities are floundering about, trying first one thing and then another, hoping that something may prove to be of value. But without a knowledge of cause, there is nothing constructive that they can do. To remove the colon as a last resort certainly does not remove the cause of the suffering. It seems to be an open confession of failure.

It is essential to understand that irritation is absolutely innocent of the taint of malignancy, hence there is no reason why it should not be remediable. Malignancy is the ending, not the beginning of the pathological process. Those who carry out the instructions given for mucous colitis will not evolve ulcerative colitis.

29

Psoriasis and Eczema

A college youth in his twenties—with all the high ambitions of the average young man—found himself forced to face a situation apparently beyond help. His entire body, his limbs, his neck, his face were covered with a mass of scaly eruptions. The scientific name for the skin trouble is psoriasis. He had been afflicted for a number of years; his eye lids were covered with eruption, his fingers were covered, even his lips. He had tried all the usual "remedies." without avail. X-rays, salves, ointments, cortisone and other drugs had proved to be of only brief help if any at all. The physician asserted, "We are doing everything we can. There simply isn't a specific cure."

Year after year, this patient with psoriasis was treated by skin specialists, otherwise called dermatologists, and all their treatments led to nothing but more inflammation and disfigurement.

The patient turned at last to a wild non-medical question: Would fasting help? Investigating, he was told: "It might." As a result, the youth journeyed to an institution that cares for clients with fasting and other nutritional measures.

He was placed upon a fast and given daily sun baths. Under such circumstances one may almost watch the melting away of the skin disease and the restoration of a clean skin. Within weeks this young man's skin was clear. He could look in his mirror again; he could face the world happily.

The human skin, the largest organ of the body, ranks with the liver and the brain in the number and versatility of its functions. A highly complex organ containing nerves, blood vessels, glands, pigment cells and fat, this waterproof and gasproof structure invests the body like an envelope, standing between the delicate inner organs and the external environment. It is the body's radiator and air conditioner, regulating through sweating, the temperature of the body, and in the same process helping to maintain water balance in the body.

To a slight extent, it excretes waste. Its pigment protects against an excess of the sun's rays. Using the sun in the process, it manufactures vitamin D. It stores fat and blood, and is the largest sense organ of the body, nerve endings in the skin enabling us to feel heat, cold, pressure, all the sensations of finger-tip touch.

Commonly abused in a variety of ways, the skin is essentially a vital organ. It is subject to a wide variety of *diseases*, the greater number of them being inflammations. Inflammation of the skin is called *dermatitis*.

The skin is fed by the blood, not from any form of exterior feeding. There are no skin foods other than the blood itself and all money spent for so-called "skin foods" is wasted. The skin as the body's protecting envelope, comes in contact with many outside substances and influences that are harmful. It is damaged in a variety of ways. Fortunately its powers of self-repair are great, so that few of these damages leave permanent marks. Most skin diseases are due to systemic causes. It is these that should concern us most.

Dermatitis may appear in myriad forms, giving rise to diagnosis of the various forms of eczema, psoriasis, dermatoses and a host of others. So far as the layman is concerned, the fine-spun diagnoses and descriptions have only short value; at best they represent merely slight variations of the same condition. Dermatologists who use only salves and internal "remedies" do not really *remedy* these inflammations.

Many cases are the results of a general or systemic toxemic state; many others are the results of taking such drugs as arsenic, mercury, iodine, potassium, and the so-called vegetable blood remedies. Some of the irritation is the result of vaccines, serums and other drugs. In all of them recovery hinges upon removal of the cause; this no salve can do.

It is not unusual for dermatologists to advise against bathing in many of these skin eruptions, as soap and water are supposed to aggravate the condition. Soap may do so, but not plain warm water. Indeed, cleanliness is half the victory in almost all of these conditions and to go unwashed is to intensify the trouble.

In all skin eruptions, even the worst forms of eczema, I insist upon frequent bathing with warm water. It may seem strange, but in many instances cleanliness is all that is required to enable the patient to get well. A few baths and the skin disease vanishes. It reminds one of bathing seven times in the Jordan that we read about in the Bible.

In all skin eruptions, diet requires first attention. Almost certainly the patient will be found to be overeating. It is common that a redundancy of starches and sugars in the diet gets a major share of the blame. In most cases the combinations are such as to favor indigestion. There is the habit of taking starches and proteins at the same meal.

This is often enough to cause indigestion and result in skin inflammation. If there is a history of drug taking, this must be given due consideration as there are many drugs that cause skin eruptions. Brome acne is a common example. Bromine is given in many conditions and is contained in many different drugs in common use.

Psoriasis is characterized by small spots, a little elevated from the surface and covered with a flaky, bran-like covering which peels, especially in hot weather, leaving the surface red and irritated, and the skin somewhat thickened.

These spots range from the size of a pea to that of a dime. Then they develop on the face, they appear much worse after shaving. They often cause much humiliation to those who develop the disease on exposed regions of the body. I recall a beautiful young girl whose psoriasis was hidden when she was in a street dress but very apparent in a bathing suit. A good swimmer, she had to give up swimming because of the humiliation brought on by this condition.

Large surfaces on the body may be involved. On the lower extremities the whole leg may be covered. In some cases the dry scales flake off at a mere touch. Psoriasis is a very persistent disease and patients suffer with it for years. It may develop only on the forearms or about the elbows, or it may cover the whole body. It tends to get better in the summer and to grow worse during the winter months.

It has a tendency to recur after the skin is perfectly clear. Indeed, it seems that to completely recover from the disease almost always requires an extended time. Slight indiscretions in eating and beverage drinking will cause a recurrence. It, therefore, becomes necessary for the psoriasis patient to live very carefully for an extended period in order to eliminate a recurrence. As imprudent eating seems to affect the condition more promptly than any other self-indulgence, it is especially important that careful attention be given to the eating habits. Even an occasional short fast, as the eruption tends to recur, is often necessary.

Eczema—early generations knew it as tetter—may develop on almost any surface of the body, but seems to occur most often on the elbows, about the fingers and wrists, on the back and on the ears, on the anus and genitals. It also develops quite frequently on the face and on the abdomen. The skin tends to thicken and crack and there is considerable itching, causing much scratching which only aggravates the trouble. The dry patches about the elbows, knees and ankles are specially prone to itch and burn.

Wrong eating plays a dominant role in the production and maintenance of this skin inflammation. It is essential in these outbreaks that correct diet follow a preliminary fast. The fast hastens the healing of the eczema. The disease is often seen in infants, where it appears to be more persistent than if it develops later in life. The fast of the infant must be conducted under the most careful supervision and only by those fully trained and competent to conduct it.

Often a long fast is not needed, but if the condition is serious, it should be taken. In some instances, a series of short fasts with careful feeding between fasts can be made to serve.

The patient should force himself to keep his hands away from the itching surface, to avoid rubbing and scratching, as both these processes tend to aggravate the condition. Cleanliness is the chief need to prevent great itching. Frequent bathing with warm water is essential. Often, indeed, cleanliness is all that is required for complete recovery.

The prostate gland is an auxiliary of the male reproductive organs. Neatly tucked around the neck of the bladder, just under the body of this organ, the utrethra or tube through which the urine flows from the bladder, passes through it. The prostrate gland secretes a fluid that is mingled with the semen after it reaches the urethra. Because of its location about the urethra its enlargement results in more or less blockage of the flow of urine.

Enlargement of the prostate is almost as common in men over thirty-five years as enlargement of the tonsils in children. For every woman who suffers with uterine disease, there is a man who has enlarged prostate, irritation, inflammation and ulceration of the urethra, and the neck of the bladder. In large numbers of men over fifty, there is more or less ulceration of the urethral portion of the prostate gland.

These conditions can be the source of much annoyance and suffering in men. It is a common cause of retention of the urine and fouling of the bladder often giving rise to discomforts in the back, hips and legs, and sometimes causes lumbago and sciatica. The irritation resulting from retention of the urine ultimately leads to cystitis (inflammation of the bladder) and even to ulceration of the bladder and its neck.

Indeed, it may not be an exaggeration to say that prostatic disease, and its influence on neighboring organs, causes more than half the discomforts of men past fifty. Many of the diseases of elderly men, for which they are being regularly and unsuccessfully treated, are but reflexes of genito-urinary disease, of which prostatis or inflammation of the prostate gland is the primary disease.

Prostatic enlargement may begin early, at thirty five or sooner, or later, even after seventy. Fat men with large abdomens and sedentary men are more liable to prostatic enlargement, as both the fat and the sedentary life interfere with pelvic circulation, the resulting blood stasis being, perhaps, the principal cause of the prostatic enlargement. Thin men and physical workers are not, however, exempt from the disease.

Enlargement of the prostate gland results in the retention of a portion of every urination—residual urine. The pressure upon the urethra and mouth of the bladder exerted by the enlargement prevents the bladder from fully emptying. A slight retention is caused by a slight enlargement of the prostate. As the enlargement increases, the amount of urine retained is also increased.

One of the annoyances of men after middle life is slow micturition, soon to be followed by a slowly developing obstruction to the flow of urine. At fifty-five to sixty there develops small retention of urine, which means that after all the urine has been passed that can be passed, there will be an ounce or two of urine left in the bladder. The inability of the bladder to empty itself slowly increases. As the same time the amount of urine retained increases. The retained urine poisons the bladder, and in, time, the entire system, causing much discomfort and suffering, even death.

As the prostate enlarges, its weight pulls the bladder downward thus making it even more difficult for the bladder to empty itself. As retention increases, the bladder becomes more sensitive and the difficulty of urination increases. Cystitis, inflammation of the lining membrane of the bladder due to residual urine, caused in turn by retention from prostatic enlargement, is quite common in elderly men. Urethritis—inflammation of the lining membrance of the urethra—also results from the irritation.

The membranes, these inner skins that line the bladder and urethra, are mucous membranes and resemble the membranes lining the nose, mouth and throat. Hence, when these membranes become inflamed, we have a profuse flow of mucus or what is commonly known as a catarrhal condition.

Long and continuous inflammation of the neck of the bladder ends in ulceration with slight hemorrhage, so that bleeding is sometimes seen, although this is not a common development. Cancer rarely occurs in this condition. When the irritated tissue has hardened it has taken the first step along the road to cancer. Cancer of the prostate is not an uncommon condition, but it is rare compared with the number of cases of enlarged prostate that develop.

Physicians say that the cause of prostatitis is unknown. We see in it another development out of wrong life. Excesses in eating and drinking and in sex seem to be the most common causes. Because no attention is given to these phases of the living habits of the sufferer, the condition tends to grow progressively worse.

I recall a conversation I had with a man who suffered with prostatic enlargement but three years ago. Describing his symptoms to me and the medical treatment he was getting, he added, "I eat like a horse." His physician had not instructed him about his eating, but was content to try to palliate his discomforts with drugs and X-rays.

No satisfactory palliation for prostatic disease had been evolved. Operations to remove the gland or part of it, injections to shrink the gland, and all other treatments that have been tried, have proved to be highly unsatisfactory.

Why? Because there are no treatments that antidote wrong life. The manner of living that results in engorgement and enlargement—also called hypertrophy—of the prostate gland cannot be counteracted by drugs and surgery. It will be necessary to correct the way of life.

When enlargement of the prostate and strangury (drop urine) have evolved, with their pain and regrets, a good surgeon can end the patient's misery—permanently. Thousands have died as a result of prostatic operations. Perfect drainage is required for a successful operation on the prostate gland and this is not possible.

For this reason, when a surgeon assures you. "The operation does not amount to anything; you'll be up and out in three days," it would be well to ask him: "Out where?" All too often it is out in the cemetery.

At present the better surgeons do not like to remove the prostate. Walter C. Alvarez, M.D., says of this: "For myself I would have only one type of operation performed, and that would be the transurethral, which is perfomed through a ligated tube which is passed down through the urethra.

"The only difficulty with this operation is that it requires much skill, and when much prostatic tissue has been removed, the urologist must be able to operate with speed."

With all the skill and speed the urologist may be able to exercise, the operation is still mere palliation. It removes no cause, it restores no health. When cause is untouched it continues to build more trouble.

At one time operations on the prostate gland were more popular than they are now. The loss of popularity was due to the high death rate which seems to have been about twenty-five percent, and to the great aftermath of trouble. The man who has an operation for enlargement of the prostate and survives the operation has not settled his account with nature. Indeed, the resort to surgery almost guarantees that he shall not be restored to health.

A troublesome prostate is the result of continued practice of habits that no self-respecting man will continue after he has learned the truth. From the systemic and not merely local effects of these bad habits, surgery can provide but temporary relief.

Prostatic surgery is intended to enable ignorant old men to side-step the results of breaking the laws of biology in their mental and physical habits. To give up the physical and mental bad habits that build prostatitis will enable these patients to get well, providing the change of habits takes place early enough.

Advanced prostatitis is a condition that can be completely remedied only in a small percentage of cases, but those so afflicted can be taught how to live to make their lives more comfortable and to greatly prolong life. Once the prostate gland has enlarged, there seems to be a strong tendency for it to enlarge again on slight provocation. Even after it has been brought down to normal size, it re-enlarges with ease and speed if the patient does not rigidly adhere to a healthful way of life.

I have seen prostate glands that were as large as baseballs and nearly as hard—cases in which a catheter (an instrument used to draw off urine) had been inserted and used because the passing of urine was a painful process. The enlargement was reduced to nearly normal size in a week, the hardness was entirely dissolved, so that urination was normal after proper care was given. Commonly, however, more time than this is required to reduce the prostate.

In some cases it does not seem possible to reduce all of the enlargement, but it may be reduced so that the urine flows freely, all discomforture in the back, hips and legs (and sometimes lumbago and sciatica, which are not present all the time) are relieved. This is all accomplished by stopping enervating habits, putting the patient to bed and stopping all food.

Men who have prostatic enlargement are forced to get up frequently at night to pass urine. The irritated bladder will not retain urine in a normal manner. The nightly promenading interferes with sleep and this results in further eneveration.

I have seen these patients who were forced to be up as many as fifteen to twenty times a night. I have seen them, after a few days of fasting, sleep thirteen hours in a stretch without having to void urine. Men who had great difficulty in passing urine were able to do so as freely as when they were boys.

In only a small percentage of these cases is this improvement permanent. I have seen numerous instances in which the enlargement recurred within two or three weeks. Overeating will result in a speedy re-enlargment of the prostate. Nervous excitement, over-work, sexual excesses, and a variety of other enervating indulgences will do the same. Tea, coffee, tobacco, alcohol and other stimulants quickly cause the enlargement to recur.

The fast in these cases provides only temporary relief if the way of life is not changed. The engorgement and enlargement of the prostate gland may be reduced by a fast, but this is not all that is necessary to the restoration of health. A short fast is certainly inadequate to reduce the prostate more than a small amount. It will make urination easier and relieve some of the distress, but a few days afterward the trouble will be as severe as ever, unless radical, sweeping changes in the ways of life are made.

The fast may be used as a means of controlling the enlargement in those cases where it cannot be permanently eliminated. If indiscretions in eating or in other facets of living have resulted in re-enlargement of the gland, a fast of one to two days is commonly enough to restore a free urine flow and relieve the discomfort and difficulty.

This may be repeated at intervals as need arises. But no amount of fasting will compensate for the failure to correct completely the mode of life. If the way of life is not changed, fasting becomes a mere palliative and, though far less harmful than other forms of palliation, leads the individual to depend upon palliation rather than a radical correction of cause.

"I have gonorrhea; what shall I do?" The voice came over the telephone from a near-by city. The caller was advised to fast at once, with rest.

"But I have to work, my business requires my attention. I cannot fast. Would it not be better to take penicillin?"

Penicillin would suppress the symptoms he was told, but they would recur in a brief time. After a short discussion, he decided to take penicillin. A few days later he called again and triumphantly announced that he had taken penicillin, this being administered by a local physician, and that his symptoms had all speedily cleared up. It was an old story, but one that he did not understand. Several more days passed and he called again.

"The symptoms have returned," he said. "What do I do now?"

Again he was advised to fast. Again he said that he could not fast. A fruit diet was urged. He said he would try it. Eventually, after repeated failures by other methods, he went on a fast and was soon free of his symptoms with no recurrence.

"Failure Against Gonorrhea," was the significant title of a press release made in December, 1962, by the World Health Organization. The experts on gonorrheal infection of WHO reported that "in spite" of the widespread employment of penicillin and other "powerful anti-biotics" complete failure to control gonorrhea throughout the world had been registered.

Instead of wiping out the disease as the first optimistic prediction promised us, there had been for a few years an increase in the number of cases. They estimated that there are 60,000,000 new cases of gonorrhea each year in the world, an incidence that they blame largely on the teen-agers—young people who had been taught that a shot of penicillin will "fix you up" in jig time.

Figures the Committee accumulated reveal that gonorrhea is more common between the ages of fifteen and twenty-five than at any time in the past.

Many sections of the United States have reported an alarming increase in venereal disease that is swamping clinics and control centers. Just to take the figures released in 1962 by one state, California: 26,932 cases of gonorrhea were officially reported by physicians.

Compare this with 14,697 cases reported in 1955. It is asserted that these figures for 1962 do not begin to tell the story, for although the law requires all physicians to report such cases, many fail to do so. Indeed, it is said that such cases are rarely reported. Less than ten percent according to estimates of the cases of gonorrhea have been reported. It is stated that teen agers and young adults are the chief *victims*.

The false security that was aroused by the first optimism for the anti-biotics, has now given way to despair—and alarm. Physicians admit that penicillin and steptomycin are "no longer effective" against the disease. The common explanation is employed: the germs have developed res.stance to the drug.

Even progressively larger doses are now admitted to be resulting in more "treatment failures" than did much smaller doses when the drug was first used. It is now realized that it is not possible to treat gonorrhea out of existence with universal use of anti-biotics.

While one may have gonorrhea numerous times in a lifetime, it is well known that one *infection* does not confer *immunity*, as is claimed for many other infections; it is now said by the experts of WHO that the only hope for the future resides in the possible finding of a vaccine that will confer *immunity*. It is strange that they never suggest that good behavior is a sure preventive. They take it for granted that youth has started on a course of sexual laxity from which it cannot be returned, no matter what the cost.

My observations as well as statistics of the disease show that circumcision is a very poor substitute for good behavior. The disease is very prevalent in circumcised as well as noncircumcised peoples of the world.

Before the days of penicillin I used to get numbers of cases of gonorrhea for care. Then came the "wonder drugs" and the belief that one to three shots would rapidly *cure* gonorrhea. I ceased to get these patients. Everybody who developed gonorrhea resorted to penicillin. Symptoms were thus suppressed and recurrences were again suppressed. But suppressing symptoms does not provide any lasting answers.

Gonorrhea is a self-limited disease. This is to say, it runs a more or less variable course to recovery. Patients get well under all kinds of treatment and they get well with no treatment at all. A number of years ago some tests were made and it was discovered that warm water was as effective as the drugs popularly used. The course of gonorrhea runs from four to six weeks. Its course can be shortened by rest and fasting. Complications can be prevented in all cases by fasting.

Every enervating influence, such as tobacco, alcohol, overeating, lasciviousness, late hours, over-activity, will delay recovery and increase the liability to the development of complications.

My own experience has indicated that the disease gets well more rapidly in females than in males and there is less suffering, due primarily to the fact that the female canals are larger and drain better. Adequate drainage is vitally important and any bandages or ligatures that interfere with drainage are almost certain to cause complications.

This is one condition in which I think that we may profitably alter our rule against drinking much water, and permit the free taking of water. Much water drinking means frequent urination and this helps to keep the urethral canal washed out. Injections into the canal tend to carry infectious material further back into the canal, whereas urine tends to sweep it to the mouth of the urethra and out. Externally, both in males and females, strict cleanliness is essential.

While I prefer the fast in all such cases, if the circumstances of the patient are such that a fast of any length is not feasible, the fruit diet may be substituted for the fast. Three meals a day of fresh fruits, with no eating between meals and no heavy fruit meals taken, will enable the patient to carry on his activities and get will without complications.

Fasting or a light diet of this kind not only hastens recovery and prevents the development of complications, but it also assures the patient greater comfort while the disease is at its height. There is less pain and in the case of the male, fewer painful erections.

Again, I emphasize: the fast is not a *cure;* it does not *cure* gonorrhea. The self-healing processes of the body eliminate the cause of the gonorrhea and restore the normal state. When one fasts under such conditions, one merely avoids putting hindrances in the way of the reconstructive processes of life.

32
Paralysis Agitans

A woman nearly forty years old arrived at a *Hygienic* institution in this country, a fter suffering with Parkinson's disease for six years. Her home was in Costa Rica, her husband was an Austrian engaged in the importing business. When her first symptoms appeared a physician was consulted. After a few local physicians had been given the opportunity to restore her to health, her husband took her to Vienna, where she was given the best medical care Europe afforded at the time.

Two years later she was brought to New York, where she was again treated by the best specialists on the east coast. After a total of six years of the finest care available, with no results except that her condition had grown progressively worse, she was taken to the *Hygienic* institution.

At this institution she was put to bed and placed upon a fast. As progressed, she gained control of her limbs. After a fast of more than thirty days, she was allowed to resume eating. There was an immediate recurrence of tremor, but it was not so bad as before the fast. The results were the same, except that the tremor was much less, after the second fast as after the first.

After another period of eating, she was given a third fast. There was no recurrence of tremor afterwards. For more than ten years, thereafter, as long as the *Hygienist* was able to maintain contact with her,she had no recurrence of the tremor. She carried on the work of her household and enjoyed better than average health. The total time during which she was under *Hygienic* care was nine months.

The developments in this case are typical, with the exception of the completeness of recovery. Not all cases make full recovery; indeed, full recovery is not the general rule. The rule is that the majority of these cases make sufficient progress to become useful again, but retain a part of the tremor.

There are a small number of cases, in late stages of the disease, that make no appreciable improvement. It is correct to say that cases that make full recovery and cases that make no improvement are both comparatively rare. This is apparently true for the same reason in both instances: *Hygienic* care is instituted much too late. It is rare that a patient with paralysis agitans undergoes *Hygienic* care at the first appearance of symptoms. Indeed, the author has never known of such an instance.

Paralysis agitans, also known as shaking palsy and Parkinson's disease, was named after Dr. James Parkinson, who was British. He first described the disease in 1817. It commonly develops late in life, usually after the age of forty. It is slightly more prevalent in men than in women, and is characterized by stiffness and rigidity of the muscles, which causes delayed action of the voluntary muscles, and by tremor, which is chiefly noticeable when the patient is sitting still and disappears when he is active. A description of a typical very advanced case reads: "Quaking of the limbs, rigidity of the muscles, an abnormal slowness of movement, staring wild-eyed without blinking, right facial expression, and often drooling from the mouth."

There are an estimated 280,000 cases of paralysis agitans in the United States, with thirty-six thousand new cases developing each year.

Tremors, whether coarse or fine, result from alternate contraction and relaxation of opposing muscles. They are not confined to paralysis agitans, but are seen in cases of venereal excess, chronic alcoholism, delirium tremens, opium, chloral, mineral drug and other forms of poisoning. They may also be seen in many cases of neurasthenia, debility, senility, arteriosclerosis, hysteria, goiter, paresis, etc.

Usually affecting the hands and feet, the tremor of senility is exceedingly fine. In paralysis agitans the tremor is rhythmic and regular and persists during sleep as well as during waking hours.

Beginning mildly, paralysis agitans progresses gradually with tremor and weakness beginning in an extremity, usually one hand and arm. In the beginning the tremor can be controlled by the will, but the disease gradually extends until an entire side is affected and it becomes no longer possible to control the tremor.

In advanced stages, there is often dullness of the mind, drooling, a tendency to go forward (the so-called propulsion walk), and restlessness of the fingers, which appear to be continually going through the motions of crumbling bread. There is a progressive loss of power in the affected muscles, moderate rigidity, alternations in the gait, and, at times, mental impairment. In advanced states, the tongue and chin may become tremulous. Rarely is speech lost. Some of the patients become very much worse under excitement and so great is the tremor that they literally jump up and down.

Often the tremor is of minor importance in the estimation of the patient. He visits a physician for hypertension, digestive troubles, arthritis or other affection. I have seen one or two cases of arthritis, with rigidity of the limbs, in which the tremor showed up only after the arthritic condition cleared. The arthritis seems to have masked the paralysis agitans.

Wilson's disease so greatly resembles Parkinson's disease that it is difficult to distinguish them. In Wilson's disease there is also enlargement and sclerosis of the liver. In general, Wilson's disease would seem to be less favorable than paralysis agitans. It appears to be much rarer.

The single case of a woman I have seen personally did make considerable improvement during a period of three months under my care. She had been unable to write for seven years, so great was the tremor of her hands and arms.

After two weeks of fasting she was able to write letters and was able to hold her hands as steadily as the most normal individual. There was a recurrence of tremor after the fast was broken, but it was not great enough to prevent her from writing letters. No second fast was undertaken and the patient passed from under my care.

Paralysis agitans is defined as a "nervous disease of unknown origin." Its cause is said to be "entirely unknown." Studies of changes in the brain and nerves all follow the death of the patient, hence the findings represent end-points rather than the condition of these structures at the first appearance of symptoms.

Patients often live for as many as twenty or more years after symptoms first develop, so slowly does the disease progress. Certainly the changes in the brain and nerve tissue at the end of a twenty year period of development tell us nothing of the condition of these tissues twenty years earlier.

It is not enough to say that sometimes the nervous system wears out prematurely; it is essential that we trace the cause of the premature wearing out of the brain and nerves. What is the cause of the premature wearing of these vitally essential tissues? In later life paralysis agitans is supposed to occur as a result of hardening of the arteries which supply the nerve cells at the base of the brain and which have an important office in controlling the muscles of voluntary motion.

Or it may develop rather early in life as a result of degeneration of the brain cells themselves. In a few instances it has followed a head injury.

Often tremor is seen in men of great enervation, especially in men past sixty, in whom hardening of the arteries is already well advanced. Tremors often put in their first appearance after some exhausting experience that leaves the individual profoundly enervated.

It would seem that the causes of great enervation and of tissue hardening are the most likely reasons for paralysis agitans. Among these sexual excesses are probably of great importance.

Enervation is brought on by overindulgence in the pleasures of work and play—over-enjoyment of the wholesome activities of our existence.

Ambition, as much as necessity, can drive a man to overwork. The desire to make money, to have money to spend, is a driving force in the life of many people that causes them to burn the midnight oil. Overeating, sexual excesses, indulgence in the various poison-vices, emotional unrest, lack of rest and sleep—these and many other enervating influences in the life of man bring on a state of nervous fatigue.

Manganese poisoning will produce tremors and there is some evidence that spinal irritation, as seen in spinal curvature, may sometimes enter into these cases causitively. Tremor is said to have been a common aftermath of *encephalitis lethargica*, a disease that is very rare today, except as an aftermath of smallpox vaccination.

Medical authorities say that there is no remedy for paralysis agitans. In general, I agree with this verdict. But I have had recoveries apart from medicines, drugs or surgery, and I have seen so many cases make marked improvement during the course of a few weeks to a few months, that I am convinced a majority if not all cases could recover if proper care were instituted at the first sign of symptoms.

I have never had an opportunity to care for a case from its beginning, but have received all such cases after they were considerably advanced and had been drugged for three or more years. The drugs employed to control the tremors undoubtedly further impair the brain and nerves.

Cases following head injuries (traumatic cases) and those following *encephalitis lethargica* are less favorable cases, but in non-traumatic cases, excellent results may be obtained in the great majority of patients in a comparatively short time. But full recovery, where possible, is a matter of months or even of years.

It is not uncommon to see the cessation of all tremor in the first fast, only to have it recur when eating is resumed. The tremor is less severe when it recurs after the fast. A second fast produces the same results, with less tremor following this. A third fast is sometimes enough to result in a lasting clearing up of the tremor. In some cases a fourth and even a fifth fast is required.

It is impossible to say what percentage of these cases, especially in younger subjects, could make a full recovery if they persisted long enough, but we rarely expect more than marked improvement in men and women nearing or past seventy, who have had the disease for several years.

Eating between the fasts in these cases must be limited. The diet should be composed largely of fresh fruits and fresh (perferably uncooked) vegetables, with nuts or an unprocessed mild cheese for protein. Bread, animal foods, rich viands, salt, condiments, coffee, teas, cocoa, and similar beverages should be avoided completely.

All alcohol, smoking and other use of tobacco should be avoided. An abundance of rest and sleep are specially important. Sun baths are helpful, but should not be indulged to the point of enervation. I make it a practice of giving these patients light exercises—movements requiring skill rather than strength in their performance—as soon as they are off their fast.

33

Nephritis

"Your child has six weeks to live; we can do no more for her." The voice was that of the physician who acted as spokesman for several physicians who had taken part in a consultation. The place: a modern hospital.

The little nine-year-old girl who was the subject of the decision was suffering with nephritis. She had been in the hospital for about two weeks and was bloated from head to foot with an accumulation of water (dropsy), a development that is characteristic of advanced stages of this disease. As far as they were concerned she was finished—a nine-year-old nothing.

The parents of the child were not willing to give up. People are like that; they cling to hope, and do not always accept a death sentence of this kind as final. The mother suggested taking the girl from the hospital and trying elsewhere. The physician said: "You are free to take her anywhere you wish and try whatever you think may help. We can do no more."

The girl was removed from the hospital, but no other physician was found who would take charge of the case.

Taking the child on her lap, the mother sat in the back seat of the car while the father drove a hundred-and-twenty-five miles to a *Hygienic* institution. Arriving there, the father carried the child inside and presented the hopelessness of the case to the director.

"I cannot promise much," said the *Hygienist*, "but we'll try." After fully going over the history and symptoms of the case, he told the desperate parents, "We are going to give her a chance to recover. I believe she can."

The suffering child was put to bed and all food withheld. Water was given in infrequent sips. Almost over night the edema began to decline. It passed out in the urine and in watery stools, and, after a few days, some of the solid matter contained in it was expelled by means of skin eruptions. Soon wrists and ankles that were as large, or larger, than her legs were down to normal size. A little girl who looked like a rubber baby blown up to oversize was down to "skin and bones."

After two weeks of fasting, feeding was resumed. She was fed on fruits and vegetables at first, with starches, sugars and proteins added after a few days of juicy fruits and leafy vegetables. From this time forward her progress, although slow, was satisfactory. At the end of nine months the little girl was dismissed.

After the passage of several years the same little girl, now married, again visited the *Hygienist* and was in a state of splendid health. She had developed into a beautiful young woman and was proud of her exuberant health. There had been no more trouble with her kidneys; indeed, she never experienced sickness of any nature and was holding down a responsible position.

Can we say that this recovery is typical? No. Most cases of Bright's disease or nephritis, are in older men and women and the deterioration of the kidneys is greater than in the case of this young girl, so that all patients do not recover so readily or so quickly—and some of them do not recover at all. But this case does reveal that death is not always inevitable because the case has been declared to be *incurable*.

It reveals the amazing things the body can do for itself in the way of restoration of structure and function when it is given a fair opportunity. This dying child was not "treated" into good health; she made her own spontaneous recovery without the dubious assistance of any therapeutic measure.

Richard Bright, a British physician prominent in the first half of the nineteenth century, noted that the last illness of many men was attended by the appearance of albumen in the urine or uremic poisoning. He investigated the condition of the kidneys in these cases and discovered a degenerated state that was responsible for the symptoms. Although this condition is technically known as nephritis (inflammation of the kidneys) the disease has long been called Bright's disease after the man who first described it.

Actually, from a practical point of view, we are not so much concerned about the degenerative changes that take place in the kidneys, when albumen and granular and bloody casts appear in the urine or when there is suppression of the urine. When we are confronted with evidences of uremic poisoning, instead of worrying about the nature of the changes in the kidneys, we need first to think of the living habits of the patient. Faulty, excessive practices may have caused the degeneration of kidneys and all the other organs that are involved in the deterioration.

Few chronic diseases arouse so much fear and apprehension in the patient's mind as chronic Bright's disease. Yet there is no chronic disease that so quickly improves, and from which the patient is so likely to make a full recovery as a consequence of a fast, proper feeding and general *Hygienic* care. These simple changes, however, in the way of life must be made before the deterioration to the kidneys has reached an irreversible stage.

The reason for the terror that a diagnosis of Bright's disease commonly causes is based on the fact that the cause of the disease is not removed.

Nephritis or Bright's disease does not develop, neither in the acute nor in the chronic form, in those of abstemious habits of living. It is a disease of high livers and continuous stuffers. Many drugs produce inflammation of the kidneys and those who are always drugging themselves may have to pay for their folly by evolving a serious degenerative change in the kidneys that will shorten their life.

It is well known in professional circles that today the possession of typically healthy kidneys is rare in adults. Great numbers of people who die of other diseases have been made liable to these other diseases by the impaired state of their kidneys.

A fast in this condition need not always be a lengthy one. Ten days, two weeks, sometimes three weeks, are usually enough. The condition of the kidneys quickly clears when fasting is instituted. The albumen disappears from the urine, casts and blood clear up. The symptoms of urine poisoning—headaches, vertigo, frequent and copious urination, bed wetting, getting up frequently at night, suppressed urine, and scanty urine—soon cease. The urine becomes normal in color and odor and everything points to the resumption of normal excretion.

The regeneration of the kidneys that takes place after the fast is broken will be more thorough, more complete and more rapid if the diet is abstemious and composed of fresh fruits and leafy vegetables with but moderate quantities of the heavier foods.

Onions, garlic, chives, shallots, leaks, mustard, radishes, cress and other foods containing mustard oil, which irritate the kidneys, should be omitted from the diet. Grain products are also best omitted. Flesh, meat extracts, alcoholic beverages, soft drinks, tea, coffee, cocoa and chocolate are not to be thought of for the man whose kidneys are seriously impaired. Excessive water drinking can serve no useful purpose. Give the kidneys a chance to repair themselves and they will not disappoint you.

34

Gallstones

Cholelithiasis is the term applied to the formation of stones in the gall bladder and bile ducts. These are derived either partly or entirely from the constituents of the bile, the principal element being cholesterin which precipitates in crystalline form and combines with inspissated mucus.

Although the stones can be a source of much discomfort, and in passing, may be the occasion for excruciating pain their presence is frequently unrecognized and man may live for years and die of some other disease without ever knowing he has them. They are found at autopsy in people who never complained of symptoms that led to a suspicion of stones.

Some individuals have what is termed the *lithemic diathesis,* by which is meant that they have a tendency to build concretions in the form of kidney or bladder stones or biliary calculi when their health is markedly impaired. Stones may form, in fact, in almost any part of the body—in the pancreas, in the muscles, in the eyelids, on the valves of the heart, even around the heart, and in the arteries. Gallstones seem to be more likely to form in the obese than in thin subjects, perhaps because there is a greater tendency of these obese individuals to overeat.

What is called hepatic colic is excruciating pain in the abdomen, in the region of the liver or gall bladder occasioned by the passage of a stone. Calculi may be so small that they easily pass through the gall duct, in which case they are expelled without the patient ever knowing that he has any stones.

They may be too large to move into the gall duct, in which case they are not passed. Or they may be of a size that they are passed through the duct with great difficulty, and cause intense pain. The pain starts suddenly at the instant the stone begins to be passed from the gall bladder into the cystic duct. Agonizing in character, it is transmitted to various parts of the abdomen and chest, often being felt in the right shoulder.

Or the duct may be obstructed by a stone and a few symptoms result, even jaundice being absent. Disease of the gall bladder itself may eventually result from the presence of the stone. If the common duct is obstructed by a stone, there is persistent jaundice, paroxysms of pain, with the occurrence of ague-like periods of chills and fever. Often called a gall-valve condition, this may persist for months or years.

Pain killing drugs and operations are the common modes of treating this condition, but neither of these remove basic causes. To remove a gallstone and pronounce the patient *cured* is tantamount to saying that the gallstone is its own cause.

Failure to remove the cause results in the formation of more stones. Unfortunately, it is assumed that the cause of gallstone is unknown, so that the operation leaves the patient still sick and still manifesting many of his symptoms.

What is wrong with the person who has gallstones? He has a general state of irritation and inflammation of his digestive tract, involving the gallbladder and the liver, with impaired digestion. He is enervated and toxemic. His bile is not of normal constitution and this permits the precipitation of its mineral elements. There develops a functional impairment of the liver.

This persists until there is enough alteration of the normal secretion (bile) so that the mineral elements contained in this are not held in suspension, but are precipitated, forming gravels or stone. Gallstones and kidney stones are basically the same. The symptoms differ as the organs in which the stones form differ. Organs lend individuality to symptom-complexes.

Imprudent eating and heavy eating of carbohydrate foods by the enervated and toxemic, and a lack of exercise, are chief among the causes that produce gastrointestinal and biliary irritation leading to stone formation. They do not develop in healthy individuals, but in those who have broken down their health by years of wrong living. Nobody would ever have gallstones from infancy and throughout his life if he lived right.

There can be but one way to restore health and this is to remove all causes of disease and restore the liver to good health, after which normal bile will disintegrate the stones. The proper care is to go to bed and relax, keep the feet warm and abstain from food until there is a distinct demand for food—until the return of hunger.

When eating is resumed, it should be restricted to uncooked fruits and vegetables for a week or two weeks. The patient should be carefully restricted to proper food combinations when regular eating is resumed.

Eating proteins and starches at the same meal is a prolific source of gastro-intestinal irritation.

In my opinion there is no necessity to operate for gallstones. Normal nutrition is not restored by removing an effect of impaired nutrition. The great and growing army of postoperative invalids attest to the fact that operations on organs of the body do not restore health. Too many organs are removed that could be saved by the simple expediency of draining them by means of the fast.

Instead of surgically draining the gall bladder, a fast will enable the body to perform an excellent job of drainage and do it in a way to leave the gall bladder intact and unharmed. For days and nights, often, these patients will pass bile through the bowels and by vomiting.

The patient has not been restored to health when his gallstones have been removed. The observing individual knows that he is still sick and still manifests many of his old symptoms and often many new ones. The purpose of correct care of the patient with gallstones is to restore normal liver function so that bile chemistry may become normal again and cease precipitating the mineral elements and thus end the making of stones.

In a few weeks then, the normal bile will cause a disintegration of the stones already formed, the sand will pass into the intestines and will be voided. As the liver cannot be restored to health without restoring the whole body to health, no treatment directed at the liver will serve these ends. A general or systemic housecleaning followed by a genuine health-building program is essential.

Perhaps I can do no better than end this chapter with a quotation from Geo. S. Weger, M.D., who had an extensive experience with gallstones, both as a regular physician and as a *Hygienist*. He says: "Given proper assistance, the chemistry of the body can be so altered that stones soften, disintegrate, and pass out with but slight discomfort. We have treated many cases and seldom have we found it necessary to resort to surgery. It is a remarkable fact that this softening occurs very rapidly on a complete fast. Frequently patients coming for treatment for different ailments develop hepatic colic from the eighth to the tenth day of fasting.

"In these, the presence of gallstones may never have been suspected. The same is true of stones in the kidneys. In recurrent attacks there is no treatment in the intervals to equal a diet restricted to fresh fruits, salads, and cooked non-starchy vegetables. It can be safely predicted that there will be no recurrence in those patients who follow instructions as to diet and exercise. In most instances if the gall stone is not larger than a small olive it will become soft and pass out without resort to surgery and its consequent risks. The exceptions are in those run-down people who have no reserve vitality or courage left to sustain them for a reasonable time, while nature is establishing a normal chemical balance.

"Extreme caution and conservatism on the part of the physician is necessary in determining the proper course in a given case. The process of recovery may seem slow but it is in reality marvelously rapid compared with the long time it takes for the stones to form. While most cases can get well by fasting and dieting and while such treatment is always in order, it must be borne in mind that atrophy or gall bladder disease may be the result of longstanding, unrelieved cases. Without recourse to olive oil, bile salts, and the hundred and one remedies that are generally prescribed, our percentage of non-surgical recoveries is so high as to warrant a favorable prognosis if the patient cooperates in the removal of first causes. It should be borne in mind that while surgical interference is often the only recourse, this procedure does not remove the cause of gallstones nor prevent recurrences. Therefore correct diet and other accessory health measures are just as necessary after operation as they were before."

35

Tumors of the Breast

One of those rare young women, possessed of great beauty of form and features, just married and alarmed about a growth of her left breast—a lump nearly as large as a billiard ball—had for four months suffered considerable pain. She had not consulted a physician for fear he would pronounce it cancer and want to remove her breast.

It was 1927 and that year the country went through the first "cancer week." New York's newspapers carried columns each day about cancer and urged all people to see their physicians for a check-up. Lumps, moles, bleeding, loss of weight and other such symptoms were indicative of possible cancer. The propaganda was deliberately designed to frighten the public.

The young woman, whose home was in White Plains, New York, was duly frightened. She consulted a physician. He told her that she had cancer and that the breast would have to be removed immediately. She did not want to lose her breast—she did not want to be disfigured.

She consulted a second physician. He made the same diagnosis and urged immediate removal of her breast. A third physician rendered an identical verdict. A fourth was consulted with the same outcome: "The breast must come off at once."

But there was one paper in New York that did not carry the scare propaganda that was being distributed from some central source. The New York *Evening Graphic*, a Macfadden publication, often assailed for many reasons, right and wrong, refused to join in the effort to frighten everybody. The present writer had a daily column in the *Graphic*.

I devoted a column to the cancer propaganda and pointed out that many people who did not have cancer were being frightened into operations. I denounced the fear program as a crime against the welfare and sanity of the public. The young woman read my column and came in to see me.

It was eight o'clock on a Friday evening when she entered my office. I examined her breast and decided that she did not have cancer, but that she was suffering from an enlarged gland. I advised her to fast. She took the advice. I instructed her to return to me at the same time on the following Monday evening. When she came in on Monday evening she was a very happy woman, her face wreathed with smiles. I invited her to sit down and without questioning her or waiting for her to say anything, I said, "Go ahead and tell me the story."

It was a simple story, but it was a happy one. I have listened to similar stories many times through the years that have since elapsed. "When I awoke this morning," she said, "there was no pain in my breast. There has been no pain all day. This evening at five o'clock, when I went to take a bath, I said to my sister: 'I would like to feel my breast to see if the lump is still there, but I'm afraid to . . .' My sister said: 'Don't be a child, go ahead and find out.' I investigated nervously and it is gone."

I listened to the story with great satisfaction and took the note of her elation and relief. I examined her breast and found no trace of the lump. The young woman remained under my care for the remainder of two weeks and was discharged.

I had occasional contact with this woman for thirteen years after her recovery and during this period there was no recurrence of the "tumor." I have been able to maintain contact with subsequent cases for as many as twenty years and they have suffered no recurrence of their "cancers." Hers was one of two such "cancers" that fully recovered in three days.

I have seen a large number recover in a week, several more to recover in two weeks, and many to become free of their breast "cancers" in three to six weeks. I am sure that not all such cases of "cancer" find their way to me or to my institution. There must be many thousands of them who submit to operations every year, either for the removal of the lump or for removal of the whole breast.

I have seen enough of them to know that there is a wide difference between cancer and a diagnosis of cancer. I am sure that these are the only kinds of cancer" that are *cured* by early surgery.

I have never seen a case of undoubted cancer recover, no matter how cared for nor by whom. I am convinced that cancer is an irreversible pathology and that the only remedy for the condition is prevention. I am sure that it can be prevented and that this can be done by a well-ordered life, one that maintains a high state of health at all times.

I think that I should call attention to the fact that all four of the diagnoses in the case of the young woman, which I have just described, were made without a biopsy, which is a procedure of taking out some of the tissue of the lump or growth and examining it under the microscope. Each man advised an operation upon the basis of a wild guess.

The biopsy is far from infallible, often finding cancer where none exists, but it is probably far more accurate than merely feeling of the breast, at these men did. Their diagnoses may be said to have been made on suspicion. Or, perhaps they were merely floating with the propaganda tide. At any rate, they all agreed without knowing the others' diagnosis, that the young woman had cancer of the breast and that an immediate operation was urgent.

Fortunately for women, not more than one such lump out of ten thousand is cancer. Most of the lumps will quickly clear up when the mode of living is corrected. Just as fasting causes the body to use up its excess fat in nourishing the vital tissues so it causes the break down, by the process of *autolysis*, of growths or tumors (neoplasms) and uses the nutritive elements contained in these with which to nourish the vital tissues.

In like manner, dropsical swellings, edematous swellings, deposits and infiltrations are absorbed and the usable portion are used as food; the non-usable portions are excreted.

To understand this, it is necessary for the reader to know that tumors (new growths) are composed of the same kinds of tissue of which the normal parts of the body are constituted. Tumors are named according to their composition. Thus a fatty tumor is called a *lipoma;* a muscular tumor is called a *myoma;* a nerve tumor is called a *neuroma;* a bone tumor is called an *ostemoma;* an *epithelioma* is made up of epithelial tissue; a *fibroma* or fibroid is composed of fibrous tissue, etc. Being constituted of the same tissue as the normal structures of the body, when they are broken down, they yield up the nutritive material contained in them.

A woman was told that she had a fibroid tumor of the uterus about the size of a lemon, and that it should be removed at once. This meant that her womb would be removed and that during surgery reasons might be discovered for removing her ovaries.

But this would not restore health. She would still be a sick woman. Operations remove no causes. There would probably be a recurrence of tumor. She would also be a physiological cripple. Cutting into the ovaries is like cutting into the brain. The patient rejected the operation and resorted to the fast. Soon the tumor was absorbed and her organs were saved.

One case that I cared for was a woman who had a uterine fibroid about the size of a medium sized grapefruit. Complete absorption of the tumor was brought about in twenty-eight days. This was an unusually rapid rate of absorption and I have never seen it take place so rapidly in another case.

I have seen tumors in the breast, on the womb, in the abdomen, on the feet and elsewhere absorbed while fasting, and some of these absorptions have been rapid while others have been slow. One man who had a large tumor in the right lower abdomen, which had been diagnosed, by means of a biopsy, as "giant cell sarcoma" (cancer) lost all of his sarcoma in seven days of fasting. Of course he didn't have cancer, but he did have a diagnosis.

For reasons that are not yet fully understood, some tumors are not affected by the fast, but thousands of tumors, some of them of considerable size, have been completely and permanently removed by fasting. I have had the pleasure of saving hundreds of women from mutilating operations for the removal of the breast, and many more from desexing operations for removal of uterine fibroids. The process is identical with the removal of stores of fat in the tissues. There is nothing mysterious about it.

The layman who can understand how it is possible to reduce weight, losing large quantities of fat in the process, by fasting, should have no difficulty in understanding how the body may also free itself of other organized accumulations of structural materials while abstaining from food.

Just as fat on any part of the body may be autolyzed and taken up by the lymph stream to be mingled with the blood and used in nourishing the vital tissues of the organism while no food is being taken, so other tissues may be digested in the same manner and used as food. Muscular tissue, glandular tissue, and other tissues may be called upon to supply nutriment for the more vital tissues, those that have to carry on the most essential functions of life.

In like manner, the tissues that make up a tumor (neoplasm) are digested and absorbed, the usable portions employed in nourishing the vital tissues, the non-usable portions excreted.

36

Sterility in Women

The pattern of the case was simple and familiar: A young Italian woman had been married for five years to a virile young man, also Italian. Both wanted children and had avoided all efforts at birth control in the hope that pregnancy would take place. It did not.

She consulted several physicians who assured her that her sterility was permanent. Her father-in-law told her of the fast and of the possibility that it might help her. She consulted a *Hygienist*.

"Will a fast enable me to become pregnant?" she asked. It was explained to her that there are different reasons for sterility and that some of them yield to the fast, others do not. After interrogation, she was told that the probability was that a fast would enable her to become pregnant.

She underwent the fast. A few weeks after the fast was broken, she conceived and later bore a bright, healthy boy.

This is one case out of many of similar nature. Fasting has enabled many women to conceive after years of sterility. Many of these women give a history of menstrual irregularities, profuse flow, severe cramps that send them to bed each month, large clots, soreness of the breasts and similar symptoms that indicate endocrine (ductless gland) imbalance, inflammation of the ovaries or womb and nervous difficulties.

Others give a history of metritis (inflammation of the lining of the womb) with a more or less chronic vaginal discharge. In these latter cases, the discharge is often highly acid, sufficiently acid to destroy the sperm.

These are the types of cases that are most readily corrected and that are restored to health by a period of physical, mental and physiological rest. Few cases of female sterility are absolute; most of them are the outgrowth of conditions of disease and are remediable. Great numbers of women have found the ability to conceive restored by a restoration to good health, and a large part of these women have found the fast of inestimable value in the clearing up of conditions that prevented conception.

In passing, it may be well to mention that in those many cases of women who readily conceive, but who abort, being unable to carry their baby to full term, a restoration of good health will enable them to give birth to normal babies. A clearing up of the toxic state followed by greatly improved nutrition enables them to avoid abortions.

The most spectacular case of this kind that has come under the author's observation was that of a woman who had previously had twenty-eight spontaneous abortions. After a fast of ten days and a period on a greatly improved diet, she became pregnant and at full term gave birth to a healthy boy. Delivery was normal.

The length of fast required in cases of female sterility varies with the condition of the woman. I recall the case of a comparatively young woman who had been married for ten years and had not conceived, although no attempt had been made to avoid it. She suffered agonies with each menstruation, going to bed every month and relieving her pains with drugs.

A fast of ten days was sufficient to permanently end her menstrual difficulties and shortly after the fast, she conceived for the first time, subsequently giving birth to a healthy baby boy. Another woman much less vigorous and sick for a number of years, took several short fasts before she conceived. Her previous period of sterility was also of about ten years duration. The young Italian woman whose story was recounted at the beginning of this chapter had a fast of thirty days.

Absolute sterility is a comparatively rare condition in both men and women and fasting can do nothing in such cases. When sterility is due to conditions of disease, rather than to defects of development, there is reason to think that both men and women can almost always profit by a fast of sufficient duration to enable the body to clear its abnormal states.

37

Fasting in Pregnancy

When the rational mind recognizes that pregnancy is a normal biological process, it at once realizes that it should be unaccompanied with any pain, discomfort or abnormal condition. It is observed that animals in their natural state do not suffer with nausea and vomiting during pregnancy. The condition is said to be unknown among so-called primitive women. Only about half the women in civilized life so suffer.

All the evidence points to the conclusion that nausea, "morning sickness" and vomiting are not essential developments during pregnancy. Mild and evanescent in the majority of the cases, severe and lasting in some cases, perhaps leading even to the artificial ending of pregnancy "to save the mother's life," the cause is still a matter of much debate.

If it can be understood that disease is the outworking of natural law, we may understand that under certain states of the organism of woman, when pregnancy occurs, there is an urgent need to put the physiological house in order.

It is common to say that the nausea is a "reflex" and that it is a "reaction," but these words explain nothing. It is necessary that we understand the nature and cause of the condition that gives rise to the "reflex" or to the "reaction."

Nature plays no favorites, is no respecter of persons. If a woman suffers with nausea and vomiting during pregnancy, this is because she has built her suffering by a way of life that has laid the foundation for trouble. Her suffering is not due to the fact that she is pregnant, but to the fact that she is toxemic.

While we recognize that pregnancy is a normal physiologic state, we must also recognize that, in modern life at least, there is much that is not physiologic associated with the whole reproductive process and that these conditions of abnormality have the same general causes that are responsible for other structural and functional abnormalities of the body.

In her efforts to promote life and its highest welfare, in her never-ending effort to endow each new form of life with the finest that can be given, nature tries to give each child that is born the best that life affords. She is, therefore, interested in the environment of the unborn child and especially in its nutrition.

The unborn child feeds upon substances supplied by the mother. If her blood is physiologically suitable to the highest interests of the evolving embryo her pregnancy will be comfortable and even pleasurable. If she is toxemic, there must evolve a process designed to prepare a better source of nutriment for the embryo. The physiological house must be put in order to the end that the embryo may have a clean, wholesome, and well balanced habitat during its intra-uterine existence.

This does not mean that the uterus alone must be made acceptable for the evolution of the new life, but that the whole body of the mother must be made ready. For unless there is systemic preparedness, there can be no local readiness.

We observe that the general metabolism of the pregnant mother is accelerated; glands that have been all but dormant awake to renewed activity, and, if the way of life of the mother is at all wholesome, her health improves. Symptoms from which she has long suffered often clear up and she appears well again. The nausea and vomiting are merely parts of this general renovating program.

The toxemic woman is declared to be unfit for the new being. The toxins that have been retained and stored in the organism until its chemistry is profoundly altered must be removed. This calls for a radical eliminating process; it demands a temporary cessation of eating.

There is rebellion in the stomach; it rejects food. The liver speeds up its excretory function. Much bile is regurgitated into the stomach and is vomited. There may even develop a psychic revulsion to food, so determined is the organism to have its way and to clean house. If we can once understand that nature is trying to provide a clean house in which to evolve the new life, we can understand the need to cooperate in the work and not to throw monkey wrenches into the vital machinery.

The suppression of vomiting by the administration of drugs, always of doubtful efficacy, seems only to make matters worse and to prolong the period of nausea and vomiting. The woman who clings to the outworn idea that she needs plenty of "good nourishing food" and persists in eating in spite of her repugnance to food, even to the sight, odor or thought of it, only adds to her discomfort and prolongs her suffering.

The physician, called to care for a case of morning sickness, tries everything, seeking to satisfy the patient's demand for relief from symptoms, until the nausea and vomiting come to a spontaneous end, but he fails to do her any real good.

It has been said that all this discomfort and annoyance constitute a rather rude, impolite and unpleasant way of asking a woman to stop eating. But it is more than just a command to cease eating; it is a process of purification. It is a means of freeing the body of accumulated toxin. The ignorant will eat in spite of the evident demand that no food be eaten, but nature gains her point in the end; she simply throws the food back. Breakfast, noon meal or dinner, it is unwanted.

When the pregnant woman feels the first faint beginning of nausea and vomiting, she should voluntarily cease eating at once. Neither she nor the child will be hurt by ceasing to eat. A prolonged fast might injure the baby, but a few days of abstinence in the early days of pregnancy, such as the woman with morning sickness will have to undergo, will help her.

She should go to bed and keep warm. She should throw off any fears she may have and poise her mind. No drugs should be taken. My experience has shown that three to ten days are enough to enable the body to put its house in order and there is no more nausea and vomiting throughout the remainder of the pregnancy.

A period of light feeding of fruits and uncooked vegetables should follow the fast for a few days before the normal diet is resumed. By normal diet I certainly do not mean the conventional diet. Pregnant women tend to eat too much. They overeat on proteins. They need the very best of proteins, but not in large quantities. Their greatest need, however, is for fruits and green non-starchy vegetables.

In ordinary cases of morning sickness three to four days of fasting are sufficient to restore comfort and enable the woman to eat without distress. I have had one case that required eleven days for comfort and digestive ability to return.

There may be severe cases that will require a longer time than this; I have simply never had such cases. But I never had a patient fail to become comfortable in a few days. There can be no reason to abstain from fasting under such conditions and at such times. Indeed, what is to be gained from eating when there is nausea, no desire for food, and when it is known that the food will be ejected as soon as eaten? Fasting is the only logical procedure under such conditions.

One Closing Word

What I have said here, in sum, is that the body has wisdom in its very cells, and can heal itself, if we will give it the chance to heal. The fast is one way of cleansing the physical self, of giving rest to the body's organs, often overtaxed by our own wrong living and wrong eating and over-activity.

I have said that there is wisdom in the fast, in rest, in quiet, in right living and right eating and right thinking; wisdom in recognizing the toxic effect of over-eating, over-tension, drinking; wisdom, indeed, in avoiding all the various poisons that so many of us put into ourselves, into our minds and our actions.

There are no medical dogmas in this book, nor is the fast itself cited as a *cure* for anything. It is only a way of rest whereby the body—this complex and tremendous organism—will have a chance to perform its self-restoration to health and well-being, without strain or interruption, in quiet and peace and healing calm.

Index

Fasting for Renewal of Life
CONTENTS

NATURAL HYGIENE PRESS
698 BROOKLAWN AVE., BRIDGEPORT CT. 06604

MORE ABOUT NATURAL HYGIENE FROM THE NATURAL HYGIENE PRESS

The Science and Fine Art of Fasting

CONTENTS

Books From Natural Hygiene Press

Exercise!
by Herbert M. Shelton
Important rules and techniques of exercising for health, strength, endurance and beauty. Written for men, women and children. Includes the Greek ideal, physiology of exercise, weight training, posture, correcting deformities, and weight control. Illustrated.

Fasting Can Save Your Life
by Herbert M. Shelton
A layperson's guide to the benefits of fasting in many of the afflictions attributable to modern life. Shows how fasting can help you normalize your weight—whether you want to take off or put on pounds—and how it facilitates recovery from both acute and chronic disease. Discusses the basic principles of correct fasting. New preface clarifies the confusion generated by the popularity of various pseudofasts.

Fasting for Renewal of Life
by Herbert M. Shelton
A complete introduction to fasting. Shows how this natural process has been used by animals and humans since the beginning. Explains how it enhances healing and brings about rejuvenation. Describes how to fast for health and how to live after the fast to maintain the benefits obtained. Index.

Food Combining Made Easy
by Herbert M. Shelton
Compact guidebook telling what foods can and cannot be eaten together for optimum nourishment and health. Shows how the inefficient digestion of incompatible foods creates disease producing poisons. Classifies foods. Gives variety of menus.

NATURAL HYGIENE PRESS

698 BROOKLAWN AVE., BRIDGEPORT CT. 06604

Health for All
by Herbert M. Shelton
A companion volume to *Getting Well*. Of special interest are articles on the fallacy of diagnosis, rational care of the sick, high blood pressure, hay fever, fasting in heart disease, and acne. Spiral bound.

Health for the Millions
by Herbert M. Shelton
Details how the body recovers and maintins health through living habits harmonious with its anatomy and physiology. A plainspoken dissertation for the layperson on the unity of the body and the effect upon health of meat, alcohol, salt, coffee, cooking, tobacco, sex, air, light, sleep and more.

The Hygienic System, Volume 1
by Herbert M. Shelton
Explanation of the basic physiological laws of human life by which the body preserves itself against harmful elements. Tells about the function and care of the glands and skin; proper and harmful ways to bathe and dress; how to care for the colon, the feet, and body orifices; how to acquire emotional control and how to have dental health. Presents fundamentals of correct use and care of the eyes (including exercises). Includes several chapters on healthful child care. Spiral bound.

NATURAL HYGIENE PRESS
698 BROOKLAWN AVE., BRIDGEPORT CT. 06604

The Hygienic System, Volume 2
by Herbert M. Shelton

The most comprehensive guide to correct food and feeding based on the findings of dietary science. Tells the reader about vegetable vs. animal proteins; organic food; denatured soil; the body's need for vitamins and mineral elements in combinations; why breakfast should be omitted; how to build good teeth; how to change to a better diet; how to select and prepare food, and how to feed in disease and convalescence. Includes information on pre-natal care, infant feedings, and nursing the older child. Hardcover.

Introduction to Natural Hygiene
by Herbert M. Shelton

A primer of the Natural Hygiene system, and the first book written by Dr. Shelton. Explains the revolutionary concept that disease is a meaningful and orderly process leading to health. Gives an understanding of disease symptoms such as fever, pain, coughing, and inflammation; describes the various stages of the disease process. Tells the reader how to prevent reaching the stage at which disease turns from the direction of health to catastrophic ill health. Explains the proper role of sex, fasting, exercise, and the mind in health and disease. Spiral bound.

Natural Hygiene: Man's Pristine Way of Life
by Herbert M. Shelton

An all-inclusive look at the Natural Hygiene system of health care from its first glimmerings in 1822 to its present day concepts. An account of its development and its validity as a complete mind and body system for staying well and getting well in all remediable cases. Includes information on iatrogenic disease, prevention of epidemics, and the historic role of women in the development of the Hygienic system. Hardcover.

NATURAL HYGIENE PRESS
698 BROOKLAWN AVE., BRIDGEPORT CT. 06604

Living Life to Live it Longer
by Herbert M. Shelton

Discussion of the human potential for vigorous longevity. Describes modern lifestyles that interfere with this potential and what must be done to reverse the situation. Cites the views of biologists and other scholars. Spiral bound.

The Science and Fine Art of Fasting
by Herbert M. Shelton

The most comprehensive and authoritative book available on fasting. Dr. Shelton has conducted over 30,000 fasts. More than 55 years of study, observation and experience have gone into the production of this remarkable book. Bibliography.

Superior Nutrition
by Herbert M. Shelton

The essentials of food, diet and related factors for the beginner. Shows that high-level nutrition involves more than food alone. Gives all aspects of correct food and eating, including meal planning and menus. Tells about fasting, child feeding, and caring for the sick without therapies.

Syphilis: The Werewolf of Medicine
by Herbert M. Shelton

The story of how medical treatment bears responsibility for the dangerous symptoms of syphilis. Combats medical propaganda on the subject. Spiral bound.

Are You a Candidate for Cancer?
by Hannah Allen

Traces the development of cancer through the stages of toxemia. Includes photos of blood smears corresponding to these different levels. Considers prevention, removal of cause, hygieneic care and applicability of fasting.

NATURAL HYGIENE PRESS

698 BROOKLAWN AVE., BRIDGEPORT CT. 06604

Fasting: Fastest Way to Superb Health and Rejuvenation
by Hannah Allen
For the inexperienced person contemplating a fast. A layperson explains what to expect and how to fast safely for maximum benefit. Corrects common misconceptions. Includes list of places to go for hygienic fasting and advice.

Homemakers' Guide to Foods for Pleasure and Health
by Hannah Allen
Encyclopedic handbook of Hygienic philosophy and living. Provides menus, recipes, and charts. Advice on storing food, entertaining, dining out, traveling, exercise, fasting, applying Hygienic principles to emergencies, and much more.

Dictionary of Man's Foods
by William L. Esser
Alphabetical guide to the foods which are most suitable for human consumption—fruits, nuts, and vegetables. Details their nutritional composition, history of cultivation, and proper combination. Includes instructions on conservative cooking. Suggestions for storing food and a week of sample menus. Special color section shows several varieties of breakfasts, lunches, and dinners.

NATURAL HYGIENE PRESS

698 BROOKLAWN AVE., BRIDGEPORT CT. 06604

The Greatest Health Discovery
Compilation from the works of Sylvester Graham, Russell T. Trall, M.D., Herbert M. Shelton and others. The story of the evolution in health care which corrected disease by changing individual living habits instead of using poisonous drugs and other harmful therapies.

Medical Drugs on Trial? Verdict "Guilty!"
by Keki R. Sidhwa, N.D., D.O.
An expose of the present day practice of medicine, the drug industry, and food technology. Discusses the lessons of Thalidomide and the Pill, the effects of drugs on different systems of the body, why drugs cannot heal, and "a new concept of health."

Toxemia: the Basic Cause of Disease
by John H. Tilden, M.D.
Summary of eminent physician's conclusions about disease. Explains the role of enervation and self-generated toxemia in disease and analyzes the germ theory. Discusses fasting, mental and emotional poise, and other ways to get well and stay well without drugs.

NATURAL HYGIENE PRESS
698 BROOKLAWN AVE., BRIDGEPORT CT. 06604

Please Don't Smoke in our House
by Jack Dunn Trop

A humorous but serious examination of the holy herb by an ex-smoker. Explores the physiological, psychological and social ramifications of the smoking habit. Outlines a step by step method for quitting once and for all.

You Don't Have to be Sick!
by Jack Dunn Trop

An engaging self-help book. The author challenges the reader to take the role of detective and search for the causes of disease and the causes of health. Distinguishes Natural Hygiene from other schools of healing. Includes a chart for rating your progress toward higher levels of healthful living.

Health Science

A montly magazine devoted to teaching Natural Hygiene, a holistic system of living in accordance with the laws of Nature to achieve optimal health. Practical information on natural vegetarian diet, exercising for fitness, raising healthy children, living ecologically, dental hygiene, organic gardening, medical hazards, foot care, proper rest, hygienic fasting and much more. Includes stories of successful recoveries, exclusive interviews, questions from readers, useful recipes, book reviews, and news.

For Other Books On Natural Hygiene Write:

NATURAL HYGIENE PRESS
698 BROOKLAWN AVE., BRIDGEPORT, CT. 06604

About the Author

No man is better qualified to write a book about fasting for health. Having conducted probably more fasts than any man now living, Herbert M. Shelton is the foremost authority on this subject today. For over fifty years, he has managed his own institution where people from all parts of the world, in varying states of health and impairment, have come to fast and learn how to preserve health.

Born in 1895, Herbert M. Shelton has been a persistent and uncompromising student and teacher of Natural Hygiene since his high school years. Though a graduate of the leading natural healing colleges of his era and possessor of several degrees, he is largely a self-educated man. Early in life, he discovered the errors and inconsistencies of all the various therapeutic systems and began to explore, on his own, the ramifications of the fact that health is maintainable only by healthful living.

A tirelessly prolific writer, he has authored innumerable articles and over three dozen books. Currently, he is editor and publisher of the *Hygienic Review*, which he began in 1939, and is still pursuing his foremost goal of eliminating peoples' fear and ignorance of disease and teaching them how they can help themselves to the health which is their birthright.